FAMILY CARE IN HIV/AIDS

D1520389

FAMILY CARE IN HIV/AIDS:
EXPLORING LIVED EXPERIENCE

PREMILLA D'CRUZ

SAGE Publications
New Delhi ❖ Thousand Oaks ❖ London

First published in 2004 by

Sage Publications India Pvt Ltd
B-42, Panchsheel Enclave
New Delhi 110 017

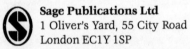

Sage Publications Inc
2455 Teller Road
Thousand Oaks, California 91320

Sage Publications Ltd
1 Oliver's Yard, 55 City Road
London EC1Y 1SP

Published by Tejeshwar Singh for Sage Publications India Pvt Ltd, typeset in 10/12 Veljovic at S.R. Enterprises, New Delhi and printed at Chaman Enterprises, New Delhi.

Library of Congress Cataloging-in-Publication Data

D'Cruz, Premilla.
  Family care in HIV/AIDS: Exploring lived experience/Premilla D'Cruz.
    p. cm.
  Includes bibliographical references and index.
    1. AIDS (Disease)—Patients—Home care—India. 2. Caregivers—India.
  I. Title.
RA643.86.I42D37   362.196'9792'00954—dc22   2004   2003027728

ISBN: 0-7619-3233-X (US-Pb)   81-7829-362-5 (India-Pb)

Sage Production Team: Leela Gupta, Proteeti Banerjee, Rajib Chatterjee and Santosh Rawat

CONTENTS

List of Tables	6
List of Abbreviations	7
Acknowledgements	8
1. Introduction: The Dynamics of Family Care	11
2. HIV/AIDS and Family Care	42
3. Contextualising the Study	74
4. Losing Autonomy and Redefining Family Relationships	86
5. Struggling to Prolong Life	107
6. Preserving Family and Learning Whom to Count on	130
7. The Way Forward	182
References	201
Index	214
About the Author	219

LIST OF TABLES

3.1 Dimensions for comparing five research
    traditions in qualitative research   76
3.2 Sociodemographic profile of participants   82

4.1 Profile of care receivers   87

5.1 Profile of seronegative caregivers   108

6.1 Profile of seropositive caregiving wives   131
6.2 Locating the spread of the seropositive diagnoses
    of caregiving wives and their husbands   161

LIST OF ABBREVIATIONS

AD	Alzheimer's dementia
ADL	Activities of daily living
AIDS	Acquired Immune Deficiency Syndrome
ARC	AIDS-related complex
BP	Blood pressure
CSW	Commercial sex worker
GPA	Global programme on AIDS
GRID	Gay related immune disorder
HAART	Highly active anti-retroviral treatment
HH	Household
HIV	Human Immuno-deficiency Virus
HRQL	Health-related quality of life
IADL	Instrumental activities of daily living
IV	Intravenous
IVDU	Intravenous drug user
LTC	Long-term care
NACO	National AIDS Control Organisation
NGO	Non-government organisation
OPD	Out-patient department
RMO	Resident medical officer
SAP	Structural adjustment programme
STDs	Sexually transmitted diseases
TB	Tuberculosis
TV	Television
UNAIDS	Joint United Nations Programme on HIV/AIDS
UNICEF	United Nations Children's Fund
USAID	United States Agency for International Development
Z$	Zimbabwean dollar

ACKNOWLEDGEMENTS

My academic interest in family care stems from my personal experience of having been a primary caregiver to my parents and husband and a supportive caregiver to my grandparents. Researching the area has helped me find answers to the many questions that crossed my mind as I performed this role, while simultaneously throwing up new ideas, insights and issues.

Family caregiving is an intensely personal experience, and I am grateful to the participants of the study on which this book is based, for allowing me into their private worlds. Undoubtedly, this called for a special sense of courage and trust since their experiences centred around Human Immuno-deficiency Virus/ Acquired Immune Deficiency Syndrome (HIV/AIDS), an illness shrouded in multiple negative meanings. Many of the seropositive participants have since passed on from this life, but it is my hope that their stories will influence the lives of those who read this book.

Committed professionals working in HIV-related service organisations put me in touch with my participants and I owe them a debt of gratitude: Sara D'Mello, Kamini Kapadia, Karen Pinto, Madhavi Shinde, Tripti Sharma, Vimal, Milan, Ratna, Agnes, Nora, Capt Pawar, Dr Nagesh, Arun, Sunny, Tony, Charlie, Manda, Capt Harish, Ignatius Vaz, Sr Lata, Sr Henrietta, Lawrence Rajnaigaum, Dr Jaju, Dr Shashank Joshi, Dr Rajiv Jerajani, Dr Nihal Mehta and Shobhana.

This research is based partially on my doctoral dissertation, completed at the Tata Institute of Social Sciences, Mumbai. I appreciate the supervision of my thesis advisor, Dr Shalini Bharat, whose exacting guidance taught me many important academic lessons.

Dr A.H. Kalro, Director of the Indian Institute of Management Kozhikode, where I currently work, has shown interest in the publication of this book. Madhu and Prasheeb's assistance with the preparation of some of the tables and Viju's contribution to the finalisation of references is gratefully acknowledged. Ashok Pathak, Manoj, Sadanand and Keshavan Nair, deserve a special mention for their support.

My husband, Ernesto Noronha, has been a real pillar of strength through various ups and downs, particularly during the writing of this book. His keen academic sense and enterprising demeanour are inspiring, and I am always amazed by his resilience. My parents set the foundation for my academic career and always remain at hand to help me whenever I require—it is difficult to find appropriate words to thank them.

I thank Debjani Dutta, Proteeti Banerjee and Roshan Thomas of Sage Publications who have been in regular touch with me during the preparation and publication of this book. Their interest and encouragement have been heart-warming.

Premilla D'Cruz
January 2004

1

INTRODUCTION:
THE DYNAMICS OF FAMILY CARE

Family care is considered to be a self-evident activity that involves assisting ill and infirm relatives. However, attempts to define this seemingly simple concept highlight the complexities involved. For instance, while Waerness (1985) defines family caregiving mainly in physical terms as custodial or maintenance help or services rendered by a family member for the well being of relatives who cannot perform such activities themselves, Graham (1983) contests this, maintaining that care goes beyond mere physical assistance. According to the latter, the provision of care encompasses the emotional aspect of managing feelings and establishing and maintaining relationships. Traustadottir (1991) distinguishes between caring for and caring about. Caring about involves affection and a sense of psychological responsibility, while caring for encompasses both the performance of concrete tasks and a sense of psychological responsibility.

Walker et al. (1995) point out that conceptualising family care as the provision of aid/assistance from one or more family members to other family members beyond that required as part of normal everyday life makes it difficult to distinguish it from aid given as part of the normal exchange in family relationships. Some of the confusion rests in the history and nature of the connection between the care receiver and the caregiver. That is, even when care receivers have similar levels of dependence, the help provided by family caregivers differs by gender and by generation. For example, caregiving husbands report giving more care than wives. The authors suggest that caregivers report activities that are not ordinary for them, or are not part of their normal responsibilities. Since many caregiving activities are consistent with everyday household (HH) work that women traditionally perform, caregiving mothers and wives may not consider such tasks to be caregiving activities; however, husbands who are less often involved with such activities and who take on such tasks primarily because wives are unable to do so, see them as caregiving. In the same way, daughters may distinguish between the tasks they do in their own homes from those that they do in the homes of their mothers. Cleaning the home is women's work, but having to do it in another's house is caregiving. Since both helpers and help recipients appear to define caregiving relative to gendered responsibilities and tasks, such subjective perceptions make defining caregiving difficult. Walker et al. (1995) hold that the criterion for caregiving should be dependence on another person for any activity essential for daily living. This criterion is based on the functional status of the care receiver rather than on the activities of the caregiver. The criterion of dependence argues that in defining caregiving, it is insufficient to ask what caregivers do; one must also ask if the family member is dependent on aid. Caregiving means providing assistance above and beyond the aid given to physically and psychologically healthy members. Under this definition, caregiving is assistance provided to someone who is dependent on that assistance.

Given and Given (1994) distinguish between two forms of assistance: direct care and indirect activities. Direct care includes the supervision of, arrangement for, assistance with, or performance of those self-care and other tasks related to physical comfort and emotional support that maintain the comfort of patients. Direct care may include personal care, pain and other symptom management, assistance with medical care activities, and emotional care. Indirect tasks include all those activities which allow the patient to remain at home and receive care there, including cooking, cleaning, shopping, money management and scheduling and transporting patients for treatment (ibid.).

Brown and Stetz (1999), in their elucidation of the process of caregiving in chronic and potentially fatal illnesses, provide further insights into the intricacies and nuances of family care. Caregiver experiences were termed the labour of caregiving (i.e., the ongoing physical, emotional and cognitive work of providing care), which begins with diagnosis and continues for several months after death. The labour of caregiving has four phases. The initial phase of becoming a caregiver focuses on adjusting to the new role, starting with coming to grips with the diagnosis and the new reality, choosing to provide care, developing competency in task performance, and alternating between hope for life and the possibility of death. The second stage of taking care involved guiding, giving and doing for the ill person to meet his or her needs. This included managing the illness, struggling with the healthcare system, managing the environment and organising resources, coming to know one's own strength, handling one's own pain, responding to family issues and preparing for death. Midwifing the death dealt with providing comfort, managing interactions and orchestrating resources during the final days. While waiting for death, caregivers continued to support and attend to their loved ones' needs. Since many of them felt that the patients' quality of life during their final days was a reflection of their competence and an ultimate expression of their love, they set the highest standards of performance for themselves. In the final stage—taking the next step following the patients' death—caregivers sought to bring closure to their caregiving role and reconnect with their own lives, a process influenced by the length of their involvement in caregiving and strength of identification with and internalisation of the caregiving role. While experiencing relief from intensive caregiving, they attempted to tie up the loose ends by completing healthcare payments, returning medical equipment, notifying insurance agencies, and so on. Dealing with regrets over past situations they wished they had handled differently, building a new life away from caregiving as well as adjusting to the absence of the care receiver were some important aspects. Brown and Stetz's conceptualisation highlights the dimensions of caregiving beyond the actual tasks involved, focusing on an unfolding trajectory that starts as an insidious, unrecognised and invisible process and ends as a central role for the caregiver.

As the preceding paragraphs show, the definition of family care should be comprehensive enough to highlight its multifaceted yet distinct identity within the spectrum of family roles and responsibilities.

Globally, family care is a topic of immense contemporary significance because of the increasing number of families with chronically ill, disabled or elderly members, who are cared for by others in the family. This trend is due to the profound changes in the way these individuals are served. While in the past long-term institutionalisation of such people was the option for families, in recent times community care is being promoted as the preferred alternative. To some extent, it is policies of mainstreaming and integration which suggest that care receivers benefit from living in a family setting located in the general population that are responsible. On the other hand, cutbacks in social welfare expenditure which make the provision of quality care for large numbers of people economically unfeasible for institutions, also play a role. As a result, individuals in need of care live in the community and are supported by their families. Progress in medical science increases their life expectancy. Medications also help such individuals to participate in many activities associated with normal people on a daily basis, with less risk of disrupting their daily routines. The family, therefore, has an expanded set of responsibilities as the interface between the affected individual and the larger society. The net effect of these trends is that the family plays a considerably more pivotal role in the care of individuals than it did in the past (Seltzer and Heller 1997).

Family care has become an active area of research in a bid to throw light on an emerging phenomenon. This book, which describes family care in HIV/AIDS through the lived experiences of caregivers and care receivers, contributes to our knowledge not only because of the contemporary relevance of family caregiving, but also because of its focus on HIV/AIDS which, being a new disease is little understood, and yet because of its stigmatising, terminal, long-drawn and debilitating nature, poses unique challenges. In the sections which follow, a review of the available literature on family care is presented to provide the reader with an idea of the field so far. An extensive survey of the literature highlighted the paucity of Indian work in the area, necessitating a reliance on Western sources. The limited Indian literature focuses essentially on the measurement of the caregiver burden, a concept discussed later in this chapter.

THE ORGANISATION OF FAMILY CARE

Family ethos is seen as the primary underlying principle behind the family's assumption of the caregiving role (Pyke and Bengston

1996). Pyke and Bengston identified individualism and collectivism as the two distinct cultural patterns within family ethos, both of which undergird different strategies of family care. In their study of elderly care, they found that since individualists are guided by obligation rather than affection, they minimise caregiving, relying on formal support in the care of frail elderly parents but maintaining regular social contact and serving as managers of their parents' finances and care arrangements. Collectivists, motivated by love and commitment, assume care of frail parents even when care demands are high, and associate nursing homes with family abandonment and dickensian conditions. Though caregiving constrains their lives, they do not resent the burdens but derive a positive identity from their role. Within themselves, collectivist families have been described as adopting traditional gender arrangements, with caregiving work assigned to women, while individualist families are seen as egalitarian.

Notwithstanding the role of family ethos, life-cycle factors also operate since different stages pose different challenges, some of which call for care seeking rather than caregiving (Aldous 1994; Given and Given 1994). Besides, Piercy and Chapman (2001) highlight the influence of expectations, family rules, religious training, role modelling and role-making in deciding how adult children become caregivers to elderly parents with functional impairments, and what roles their own children adopt in the process.

Within the family, gender determines who assumes the caregiving role. Across the globe and across the family life cycle, women remain the primary nurturers, kinkeepers and caregivers. It is the structural assumption that women's primary orientation is to the family and the extension of women's 'natural' role of mother that prescribe their role as primary caregiver. That is, the social construction of gender determines who will assume the caregiving role (Abel 1991). In other words, the term family caregiver is a mere euphemism for a primary caregiver, who is typically female (Hooyman and Gonyea 1995). Men step into caregiving roles only when women are unavailable, and even then, maintain the dominant culture's ideology that it is women who are the natural caregivers (Kaye and Applegate 1990).

The feminisation of caregiving is apparent in both its objective and subjective dimensions. The traditional gender-based division of family labour is intensified regardless of the stage in the family life cycle (Cook 1988). Cultural ideologies and assumptions about the feminisation of care are so deeply ingrained in both men and women that neither questions these beliefs (Aronson 1992). Since these ideologies create a dichotomy between feminine love and masculine self-development, they result in different ways of caring for men and women such that men's caregiver role is an extension of fatherhood and women's caregiver role is an extension of motherhood (Cancian 1987). Further, because both genders assert that housework is a woman's lot, women feel that assistance is unnecessary, while men feel entitled to support (Twigg and Atkin 1994).

Family division of labour models are advanced to explain existing gender differences in caregiving. The time available hypothesis posits that competing role and time demands restrict the amount of time an individual has for family labour. The external resources hypothesis predicts that assets obtained externally, such as income, education and occupation, determine power dynamics in the family. The ideology hypothesis states that gender role attitudes learnt during socialisation influence the division of labour. The specialisation of tasks hypothesis maintains that men and women perform different but complementary tasks in order to maximise the well being of the family (Finley 1989).

Walker et al. (1995) also cite literature to demonstrate that researchers struggle to explain how wives and mothers can continue to perform these tasks with minimal contributions from other family members and still describe their situations as fair and satisfactory. Thompson (in ibid.) has argued that women may perceive a sense of fairness in the division of household labour despite objective measures indicating otherwise, because women obtain valid outcomes from doing family work for their husbands and children. Further, women compare their situation to those of other women rather than to those of their husbands, thereby maintaining low expectations of help. Finally, women appear to accept and create justifications for their husbands' low involvement and their own overinvolvement. A compelling way to interpret the findings is to rely on gender theory. Gender theory interprets empirical information about gender from a social constructionist viewpoint. Since men and women differentially and systematically occupy certain positions in the social structure, their resulting interpretations, behaviour, perceptions and interpretations differ.

These variations, in turn, reflect the beliefs and values about gender, and simultaneously reinforce the privilege of one gender over another. According to gender theory, behaviour and roles have gendered meanings, i.e., the individual actions of women and men come to symbolise gender. Ferree (in Walker et al. 1995) suggests that women and men are engaged in a constant and contentious process of engendering behaviour as separate and unequal and of creating gender through social interaction. Since women are more often caregivers than men, and because they give more care than men, they are seen as caregivers, and this situation then reinforces beliefs about their natural propensity to nurture and simultaneously reinforces the belief that caring is unnatural for men. Thus, the power differentials between men and women are reflected in and reinforced by caregiving.

Feminists also support the social constructionist viewpoint, arguing that gender is not biologically determined. The central issue is that caregiving depends on women's unpaid and invisible labour. Women as caregivers have been historically oppressed within the home and the labour market. Being relegated to the private sphere, their lives have been made invisible and their voices silenced. They have no choice but to take on all family responsibilities, in spite of the adverse consequences. Critiquing existing policies and engineering a structural change that eliminates gender-based inequities forms an important part of this perspective (Hooyman and Gonyea 1995).

In addition to the feminised nature of family care, the literature also points to the predominance of the primary caregiver model, where one person undertakes the caregiving role with sporadic assistance from other family members (Hooyman and Gonyea 1995; Keith 1995).

Keith (1995) cautions against the overgeneralisation of the primary caregiver model, suggesting that alternatives exist where more than one person is performing the role. Moreover, the person who has the title may not be the one who actually provides the care. In his own research, Keith identified three caregiving systems: primary, partnership and team. The primary caregiver system is where one person carries all or most of the caregiving responsibilities. In a partnership, two people contribute equitably to the caregiving work and are equal in authority and responsibility. In a team, tasks are shared by a group of family members in an organised, planned and integrated manner. Factors such as family size, gender of offspring and family values were found to determine such arrangements.

Within the configuration of family relations, spouses, parents and offspring are the most likely caregivers. Spousal caregivers are the first line of defence for elders who are disabled and in need of assistance. Compared to other caregivers, spouses are more likely to give comprehensive care with less help from formal/informal support systems. In these cases, children are relatively uninvolved and the couple is more isolated. Spouses are more dependable, help with more tasks, provide more personal care and a greater number of hours of assistance, and tolerate greater disability for a longer time and at greater personal cost. Impaired elders with spouses have less likelihood of entering a nursing home. Spousal commitment is attributed to normative expectations and commitment engendered by the marriage contract. Costs associated with spousal care are mixed, with some studies reporting lower degrees of burden, and others, higher (Dwyer and Coward 1992). Parker (1994) considers the role of the spousal caregiver to be particularly stressful. The loss of a relationship between equals, the equal partner becoming a pseudo-child, the absence of support, the single-handed coping—all form relevant parts of the problem. Spousal caregivers shoulder the burden alone. Economically, they experience changes in their employment, but the fall in income is accompanied by an increase in expenditure. Socially, they are more isolated due to practical and social factors, despite their wish for companionship.

Parental caregivers include those who care for young children as well as for adult offspring with chronic illnesses and disabilities. With regard to young children, caregiving is parenting with the additional demands of having a child with chronic medical concerns (Kazak and Christakis 1994). Parents experience complex affective states including chronic sorrow, pain of outliving their offspring if the condition is terminal, and guilt if the illness has a hereditary link. While some parents cope better than others, depending to some extent on their personality, their earlier marital and family functioning, the nature of social support they enjoy and the appropriateness of medical intervention, having to care for a chronically ill child has been found to influence marital harmony, parenting styles, family dynamics, sibling development, family material resources and quality of life, and so on. Though the bulk of the literature focuses on negative outcomes, it is possible that illness could have positive impacts as well due to the increased sharing, support and self-esteem gained by the family's endeavour to master the illness (Dolgin and Phipps 1996; Feeman and Hagen 1990; Kazak 1986; Kazak and Christakis 1994; Koch et al. 1996; Ostroff and Steinglass 1996). Between the parents, it is usually the mothers who are the primary caregivers and hence the ones who experience greater strain and burden (Kazak 1986; Kazak and Christakis 1994). Fathers are more involved in financial concerns, though they may be supporting mothers in hidden and covert ways that need to be recognised and appreciated (Kazak 1986).

Parental caregiving for an adult child could be either the continuation of an earlier role if the offspring has been ill from childhood, or the assumption of a new one if the offspring's illness began during adulthood. Eventually, such caregivers form part of the geriatric population (Lefley 1996). In such instances where caregiving is endless (Milliken and Northcott 2003), and caregivers are in a state of perpetual parenthood (Rowick in Pruchno et al. 1997), parents need to reformulate what it means to be parents (Tuck et al. 1997). If caregiving is a continuation from the care receiver's childhood, parents experience cumulative burdens of their prolonged trajectory (Pruchno et al. 1997). While family social climate, income level, gender of the caregiver, nature of the illness, social support, quality of medical intervention and presence of other children to affirm one's success as parents impinge on older parents' well being as caregivers (Cook et al. 1992; Lefley 1996; McDermott et al. 1997), Cook et al. (1992) point out that the most critical variable is the ability of parents to comfort each other. Yet, despite the high burden associated with caregiving for adult children, parents prefer to provide care themselves rather than transfer it to other family members (McDermott et al. 1997). Ageing parental caregivers experience pervasive worry about the care of their children after they are gone (Lefley 1996; McDermott et al. 1997). Single parent caregivers are more vulnerable to burden and burnout since they have to deal with a chronically ill child while also taking care of other children and maintaining economic and psychological stability in the family. This is done with limited resources, including the lack of a mate with whom to share the responsibilities (Carpentier et al. 1992; Lefley 1996).

As regards filial caregivers, although affection and obligation as well as parental dependence may increase helping behaviour between adult children and their parents, conflict between them may reduce helping behaviour. The historical quality of the parent–child relationship, which may include rejection, alienation or conflict, must be considered, as it influences the willingness of children to help parents and the willingness of parents to accept help. Problems may arise if children were previously enmeshed with their parents and struggled to obtain independence and autonomy. This is so because caregiving threatens reenmeshment. It has been pointed out that even a positive relationship with parents may not lead to children providing help. Besides, a background of conflict may not only reduce helping behaviour, but may also augment abusive behaviour. The children's socioeconomic status is an important determinant of aid. Middle-class children provide more financial assistance whereas those from the lower classes give more services. Daughters, traditionally, provide more help to parents than do sons, especially in home making and personal care. Sons assist in practical matters (Blackburn 1988).

Where spouses, parents and offspring are unavailable, other family members step in. Horwitz (1993) proposes the serial model of support to explain how this happens. According to him, social support does not inhere in particular role relationships but in the configuration of the role set; if one type of member is not present in the social network, another member might provide compensatory help in their place. A hierarchy of obligations exists so that the primary basis of social support stems from the spousal and parent–child relationships. If these relationships are not available, members whose obligations do not normally include caretaking responsibilities, such as siblings, more distant relations, friends or neighbours, might assume supportive roles. Though Horwitz found empirical support for his serial model, he also concluded that sibling support does not fully substitute spousal or parental support, but is influenced by the availability of caregivers in the role set, the perception of illness severity, geographic factors, caregivers' alternative role involvement and age. Qureshi and Walker (1989) point out that the crucial role of gender in the hierarchy of obligations to elderly parents is reflected in the fact that after spouses and daughters, it is daughters-in-law who are the next lines of resort.

Finally, Given and Given (1994) cite literature to indicate that caregiving arrangements vary according to the patient–caregiver relationship. While spouses are caregivers for middle-aged patients, offspring are caregivers for older adults. In the second situation, living arrangements may be temporarily or permanently altered. Either patients move into the homes of the caregivers or vice versa. Though the conditions that dictate the direction of these moves have not been carefully documented, there is evidence to indicate that when the patient is widowed, single or divorced, multiple caregivers are involved.

CAREGIVER OUTCOMES

Though caregiving produces both positive and negative consequences for those performing it, most of the literature focuses on the negative consequences of the caregiving role for the caregiver (Berg-Weger et al. 2000; Conger and Marshall, 1998; Hooyman and Gonyea 1995; Walker et al. 1995). Indeed, Indian literature on family caregiving focuses on this aspect (Chakrabarti et al. 1995; Chandrashekhar et al. 1991; Pai and Kapur 1981; Roychaudhuri et al. 1995; Sabhesan 1991; Sequeira et al. 1990). Yet, caregivers report that they experience more positive changes than negative ones (Berg-Weger et al. 2000). While this emphasis on burden is recognised as an attempt by professionals 'to argue that families cannot absorb additional obligations and that the government must devote adequate resources to support them', Abel criticises current caregiving research 'which has focused almost exclusively on the issue of stress' (Abel 1991: 8). In her view, 'this preoccupation with stress has denied us a full understanding of the experience of caregiving' (ibid.), since it ignores the authentic connections between people, thus removing caregiving from its relational context (Walker et al. 1995). Walker et al. hold that the literature implicitly employs a social exchange theory, which posits that individuals strive in their behaviour to maximise rewards and minimise costs. Rather than focusing on net outcomes, however, there is an almost exclusive emphasis on the costs of caregiving. To be more realistic, therefore, a more complex view of caregiving encompassing both positive and negative implications for the caregiver's life is needed.

NEGATIVE CONSEQUENCES

The negative consequences of the caregiving experience have been described under the word 'burden', a concept first developed and measured by Grad and Sainsbury in 1963 (Hooyman and Gonyea 1995). Burden refers to 'the physical, psychological or emotional, social, and financial problems' that may be experienced by family members caring for a relative with a disability or impairment (George and Gwyther 1986: 253). Theoretical efforts to define the concept of burden more precisely led to the distinction between objective and subjective burden made by Hoenig and Hamilton in 1966 (Braithwaite 1992). Objective burden refers to the reality demands that confront the family member who takes on the caregiver role, whereas subjective burden encompasses the feelings aroused in family members as they fulfil their caregiving functions (Hooyman and Gonyea 1995). It is also widely acknowledged that the experience of burden is phenomenological, i.e., it lies in the interpretation of the caregiver, and hence what is burdensome to one may not be similarly perceived by another (Poulshock and Deimling 1984).

Hooyman and Gonyea (1995) provide a comprehensive review of the experience of objective burden, which includes dimensions such as the impact of the care receiver's symptomatic behaviour, deterioration in the caregiver's physical health, economic pressures, employment restrictions and reduction of leisure and social relationships. Through their review which covers a range of illnesses, Hooyman and Gonyea underscore the difficulties and constraints that caregiving engenders for the care provider. Subjectively, caregivers go through a complex mix of emotions which includes love and compassion on the one hand, and denial, shame, fear, frustration, anger, depression and guilt on the other. These feelings arise on hearing the diagnosis, in relation to the care receiver and the suffering that he/she goes through on account of the illness which brings about changes in the caregiver–care receiver relationship, in response to the challenges of caregiving and as a reaction to the extent of contribution from other family members (Blackburn 1988; Fulks and Martin 1993; Parks and Pilisuk 1991; Pratt et al. 1985; Sheehan and Nuttall 1988; Shields 1992).

DETERMINANTS OF BURDEN

Montgomery et al. (1985) and Barber et al. (1990) found objective and subjective burden to be distinct entities, poorly correlated with each other and with different correlates. According to Montgomery et al. (1985), objective burden is related to the characteristics of caregiving behaviours and the presence of helpers, while subjective burden is related to the characteristics of the caregiver. Barber et al. (1990) concluded that while both objective and subjective burden are correlated with the caregiver's health status, guilt as a result of receiving help from others, and the extent to which the caregiver perceives that others do not understand what it is like to care for a patient, objective burden is related to the number of hours of care and subjective burden to patient impairment and the quality of the patient–caregiver relationship. The predictors of subjective burden include the patient's disruptive behaviour and degree of closeness of the caregiver–patient relationship. The predictors of objective burden are the extent to which caregivers perceive that those rendering support do not understand what it is like to care for a patient, the patient's impaired social functioning, and the amount of guilt the caregiver feels when help is needed from others.

Various studies have examined the factors related to burden. Parks and Pilisuk (1991) consider characteristics of the caregiver such as age, sex, social support, locus of control and coping strategy as having a bearing on burden, while Pratt et al. (1985) see caregiver burden as related to the caregiver's support and coping but not to age, sex, income, education and patient's residence.

For Sheehan and Nuttall (1988), caregiver strain is related to patient impairment, amount of care required, affection, nature of the relationship with the patient and the caregiver's reaction to patient impairment, while the caregiver's negative emotions are linked to interpersonal conflict, level of impairment and the caregiver's reaction to patient impairment. Kramer (1993a) examined the effects of caregiver age and education; caregiver physical, social and financial resources; caregiver coping (namely, problem/emotion/relationship-focused strategies); the duration of caregiving; and patient functional status on caregiver depression and satisfaction. She concluded that poorer caregiver resources, higher caregiver age and greater patient dysfunction are associated with higher depression and lower satisfaction. The use of problem and positive relationship-focused strategies report more caregiver satisfaction but show no relation to depression. The use of emotion and negative relationship-focused strategies report greater depression but are not linked to satisfaction. Factors predicting depression include memory and behaviour problems, caregiver age, caregiver resources and emotion-focused coping. Factors predicting satisfaction comprise caregiver age, caregiver resources, problem and positive relationship-focused coping.

Boss et al. (1990) consider caregiver perceptions to play an important role in his/her experience of depression and coping. Examining this in caregivers of patients with Alzheimer's dementia (AD), they found that the caregiver perception of high boundary ambiguity (arising from the patient's physical presence and psychological absence) associated with AD hinders his/her sense of mastery and control over the situation, leading to depression and burden. While mastery is the strongest predictor of depression, ambiguity links patient functioning to mastery since it facilitates uncertainty. Severity of the illness is not related to burden and depression.

Greenberg et al. (1993) examined the relationship between subjective burden and caregiver physical health in the context of parents caring for an adult child with mental illness. The research focused on four conceptualisations of subjective burden found in the mental illness literature, viz., stigma, worries, loss and fear. The negative relationship between health and stigma and worry was significant, while that of health, fear and loss was not.

Seltzer and Heller (1997) and Hooyman and Gonyea (1995) speak of the role of contextual factors in influencing caregiver burden. According to Seltzer and Heller, four aspects define the caregiving context. The cultural context, i.e., the family's racial or ethnic group influences a lot of factors that affect the caregiving process, including how the family conceptualises the meaning of disability, the role of the extended family in providing care, the availability of economic resources and the access to the service system. The type of disability is another important factor because although there are similarities in the experiences of all parents regardless of the type of illness, there are also unique demands specific to the illness. Sociodemographic characteristics of the family such as gender and age play a role, as do the formal services families receive. Hooyman and Gonyea (1995) delineate various demographic and societal factors. The number of adults requiring long-term care has increased, largely because of the success of medical technology. Public policy advocates family care as a cost effective solution to the deinstitutionalisation campaign. At the same time, the capability of traditional family caregivers to provide care is altered due to factors such as geographic mobility, escalating divorce rates, greater public acceptance of single and homosexual lifestyles, larger numbers of women entering the workforce, growth in unemployment and underemployment, and poverty.

Dwyer and Coward (1992) highlight the gender differences in caregiving and burden. Wives care for spouses who are generally older than themselves, perceive less reciprocity from the impaired spouse and provide greater help with instrumental activities of daily living (IADL), thereby experiencing greater burden. Caregiving husbands are older, perceive more reciprocity and more help with IADL tasks from their impaired spouses, and hence experience less burden. Caregiving wives have more living children but share caregiving responsibilities with fewer formal helpers. For caregiver husbands, the greater the number of hours and the more the IADL tasks with which care is provided, the greater the burden. For wives, the greater the recipient's age, the greater the activities of daily living (ADL) impairments and the greater the number of hours of care provided, the greater the burden reported. Similarly, the greater the perceived health of the recipient and the greater the caregiver's age, perceived health and perceived reciprocity, the lower the burden for caregiving wives.

Parks and Pilisuk (1991) examined gender differences in the psychological costs of providing care to a parent with AD in relation to the caregiver's coping style, social supports and sense of control. The researchers discovered that (a) women had a higher self-report of stress than did men, although the two groups did not differ significantly in terms of depression or anxiety; and (b) women predominantly used fantasy to cope, whereas withdrawal was the more common technique for men. Perhaps more interesting is the differential effectiveness of these coping strategies for men and women in adapting to the caregiver role. Significant predictors of anxiety among the women were an external sense of control and the use of internalisation as a coping style, which predicted feelings of resentment, but internalisation was not a significant predictor among the men. For men, anxiety was predicted by lack of social support coupled with the use of either fantasy or withdrawals as a dominant coping style (Parks and Pilisuk 1991).

Literature illustrating the effects of prior marital relationships on the caregiving experience and burden leads to conflicting results where some studies indicate that good premorbid relations lower the burden while others show that they enhance it. Kramer (1993b) examined the effects of caregiver age; duration of caregiving; marital history of the caregiving spouse; caregiver's quality of prior relationship with the ailing spouse; caregiver physical, social and financial resources; caregiver cognitive appraisal of the situation; and patient's level of impairment on caregiver depression, satisfaction and quality of life. She concluded that a history of one or more prior marriages is associated with increased depression and lower satisfaction and quality of life. Lower prior relationship quality is associated with increased depression, lower quality of life and caregiving satisfaction. Lower caregiving physical and social resources and negative appraisal of stressors reported higher depression and lower quality of life. Caregiver social resources were significantly associated with caregiving satisfaction. Marital history and quality of prior relationship as well as personal resources and appraisal of stressors were predictors of depression and quality of life. Marital history and quality of the earlier relationship were the only significant predictors of caregiving satisfaction.

The quality of the caregiver–care receiver relationship is found to play a mediating role in determining whether care receiver cognitive impairments or care receiver functional impairments have a greater effect on caregiver well being. Studies show that for both filial caregivers and spousal caregivers of elderly people, greater cognitive impairment (but not greater functional impairment) was related to less emotional closeness in the caregiving dyad, which in turn was associated with the caregivers' perception of their caregiving efforts as being less effective. These results indicate that the mental, behavioural and personality changes that are typically part of cognitive impairment have a unique potential to erode positive emotional bonds between caregivers and care recipients. Consequently, the diminished positive ties between caregivers and care recipients undermine the caregivers' sense of effectiveness (Townsend and Franks 1997).

Archbold (1991), Archbold et al. (1990), Cartwright et al. (1994) and Conger and Marshall (1998) believe that mutuality, reciprocity and enrichment in the caregiver–care receiver relationship reduce burden. Deterioration in the caregiver–care receiver relationship on these counts could make burden an issue.

Caregiver burden is influenced by the caregivers' experiences with patients' relatives. Where relatives contribute little (sometimes because of geographical distance) or where they do not appreciate caregiver efforts, anger and frustration are common caregiver outcomes which often spiral into interpersonal conflicts (Medalie 1994).

The inconsistent findings about correlates of caregiving are attributed to several factors. Researchers have tended to study caregivers of people using convenience samples and have not included comparisons of groups in outcome studies. Relative to random community samples, caregivers who volunteer to participate in research may have more problems with others in their interactions. Those recruited from agencies or support groups for caregivers to people with AD are unique in that they have already sought formal care and support. It is also problematic to compare men and women caregivers because men who participate in research may be more able to give up caregiving than women who have little choice over whether to do it or not (Walker et al. 1995). Besides, across studies, different definitions and different measures of burden are used (Hooyman and Gonyea 1995).

Further, researchers have paid limited attention to the context of care, including its gendered nature, the race and ethnicity of the caregiver, the caregiver's competing obligations and commitments, and the relationship between the caregiver and care receiver (Walker et al. 1995).

In addition to burden, the caregiver as a hidden patient is another important conceptualisation. Medalie (1994) propounds this interesting concept of the caregiver as the hidden patient, based on observations of symptoms/illness/fatal diseases developing in the caregiver. He believes that these conditions are usually associated with/are the result of increased stress due to altered roles, relationships and functions, brought about by the presence of a serious, long-term illness in a close family member.

POSITIVE CONSEQUENCES

The positive consequences of caregiving have been conceptualised as caregiver well-being and satisfaction. Caregiver well-being, which refers to 'at least some periodic states of security and structure within the turbulence of life' (Goldstein 1990: 273), is associated with various caregiver and care receiver characteristics such as caregiver marital status, caregiver perceptions of their caregiving situation, caregiver personal characteristics, caregiver symptoms and the caregiver–care receiver relationship (see Berg-Weger et al. 2000 for a review). Berg-Weger et al. point out a connection between caregiver competence and well being. As the caregiver's perception of his/her competence improves, so does his/her ability to perform tasks that satisfy basic needs. Bulger et al.'s (1993) assessment of parents' appraisals of the burdens and gratifications of caring for an adult child with schizophrenia revealed that parents experienced gratification and intimacy more frequently than they did burden or conflict. While both burden and gratification were more highly associated with the caregiver–care receiver relationship than with the severity of schizophrenia or degree of caregiving involvement, even the lowest gratification scores were quite high and no subject reported a complete absence of gratification. Caregiver wives in Motenko's (1989) research associated the continuity in the closeness of the marital relationship with the perceived gratification from caregiving.

Scharlach (1994), studying employed caregivers, reported a sense of satisfaction derived from repaying elders for their previous care, enjoyment of spending time together and appreciation for help provided by the elder. In all these cases, the positive aspects co-existed with the demands of care, but the significance of these works is that unlike the singular focus of other researches, they highlighted both the problems and rewards associated with caregiving. Hinrichsen et al. (1992) underscore these observations.

The caregiving process is undertaken over a period of time, but due to a reliance primarily on retrospective self-reports by caregivers or on cross-sectional samples, the issue of how time affects the relationship between caregiving and outcomes remains unresolved. Roberto (1993) asked 48 older adults caring for ageing family members within their homes to rate changes in 14 aspects of their caregiving role over the past 10 years. The data revealed a general pattern of stability in caregiving situations over time. The most frequently cited changes were terms of physical burden (40 per cent increase), emotional burden (41 per cent increase), social activities (26 per cent decline) and financial burden (21 per cent decline). The strongest predictors of changes in the caregiving situation were declines in either the caregiver's health or the care recipient's level of impairment.

Heller's (1993) life span perspective of caregiving was based on a cross-sectional study of families grouped into five stages based on the age of the person with mental retardation (i.e., preschooler, young child, adolescent, young adult and older adult). Her data reveal that perceived burden was lowest for caregivers of the youngest (under six years of age) and oldest (30 years and older) members with mental retardation, and adolescence was perceived as the most difficult stage.

Haley and Pardo (1989), however, believe that longitudinal studies are important to account for the changing nature of stressors. According to them, longitudinal decrease in caregiver depression in cases of AD may represent successful adaptation, but may also be related to decreases in such patient problems as wandering or dangerous behaviours. Caregivers in poor health may be especially vulnerable during later phases of dementia that require direct ADL care.

As of now, two contradictory hypotheses are often posed to explain the long-term consequences of the caregiving role. The wear and tear hypothesis suggests that the repetitive nature of caregiving will take its toll and deplete an individual's physical and emotional resources. The adaptational hypothesis suggests that with experience, caregiving may get easier or become more bearable (Haley and Pardo 1989). Which of the two is a better explanation remains to be resolved.

It is quite evident that caregivers experience a variety of needs throughout the caregiving trajectory. Jeon and Madjar (1998) cite a number of research studies which highlight caregivers' needs for social support as well as for information and appropriate community and hospital services. Norbeck et al. (1991) differentiated four need categories: emotional support, feedback, informational support and exploring alternatives for the future.

More importantly, how caregivers coped with their caregiving role influenced their overall experience. Pierce (2001) found that spirituality facilitated adjustment to and acceptance of the caregiving role, notwithstanding the difficulties engendered. Spirituality allowed for a reframing of values and circumstances in such a way that caregivers felt a sense of well-being while performing this role and felt connected to their care receiving family member. While caregivers described spirituality in different ways, these expressions pointed out to love, duty and lack of options as underlying motives for caregiving.

In a study of 14 family members of people receiving hospice home care, Hull (1992) identified a series of caregiver coping mechanisms. Creating 'windows of time away from caregiving responsibilities' was important because it allowed caregivers to rest and recuperate by engaging in other activities and focusing on personal goals. Comparing themselves to others in similar situations encouraged caregivers and boosted their self-confidence. Identifying possible benefits from the situation and transforming problems into opportunities (cognitive reformation) reduced caregiver stress. To cope with the impending death, caregivers often shifted their focus to more controllable activities, for example, preparing the ill person's favourite food. Caregivers often felt uncertain and out of control, and concentrating on the present, taking one day at a time, helped them.

Langner (1993) used in-depth, focused interviews to identify three primary coping strategies used by 23 family members caring for older relatives: present orientation (taking one day at a time), retelling the reasons for caregiving (validating their actions), and establishing a routine (structuring ways to get help and respite from others). Such strategies were found to increase a sense of control and mastery for the primary caregivers.

THE CAREGIVER–CARE RECEIVER RELATIONSHIP

The process of caregiving and the development of the caregiver–care receiver relationship are inextricably linked (Himmelweit 1999). The care provided is inseparable from the relationship being developed between the caregiver and the care receiver. Through the developing relationship, the caregiver also learns skills appropriate to caring for the particular person. Other people may be able to care for the person, but in doing so, they will be developing their own different relationship. Similarly, a caregiver will have a different relationship with each one of his/her care receivers. Caregiving activities, therefore, cannot be entirely interchangeable tasks given to interchangeable people, because who is doing what for whom matters. Further, a caregiver's identity and motivation are created and developed by his/her relationship with the care receiver. Even where caregiving is initiated in response to wider social expectations, as time goes on the relationship will develop its own specific obligations and dependencies (Himmelweit 1999).

Conger and Marshall (1998) examined caregiver–care receiver relations in coresident dyads where care receivers' diagnoses were not limited by any type or category, but the latter were cognitively functional. Using grounded theory, they identified the core category of recreating life (i.e., the process of regaining integrity and pattern in biographical trajectory following a major disruption of reality caused by acute illness, which facilitates satisfactory development of caregiving relations). Conger and Marshall state that prior to the onset of caregiving, caregivers and care receivers have a relationship characterised by a particular reality or biographical trajectory that is interrupted by the illness. This disrupted reality presents uncertainty which, in order to be managed, calls for a redefinition of self and of relationship for both caregivers and care receivers. Conger and Marshall believe that redefinition of self and of relationship are core processes of recreating life, which allow for the development of new biographical trajectories. Redefining the self involves letting go and becoming. For caregivers, letting go included changing roles, grieving loss, going with the flow, living for today and focusing on the care recipient, while becoming comprised acquiring skills, coming to terms, gaining competence, gaining confidence, growing and meeting own care needs. For care receivers, letting go involved changing roles, grieving loss, going with the flow and living for today, whereas becoming encompassed acknowledging change and coming to terms. Redefining the relationship is made up of two sub-processes: collaborating and evolving, which are bidirectional and concomitant for both caregivers and care receivers. Collaborating refers to interactions between caregiver and care receiver that support the caregiving relationship. These may or may not be new to the dyad but if they were present earlier, then in their current form they are altered. Collaborating involves caring/valuing, protecting/vigilance, sharing/communicating and negotiating/compromising. Evolving occurs as dyads identify new biographical trajectories for their relationships, and is characterised by growing and bonding, altering priorities and creating shared meanings. Although redefining the relationship is a separate process from defining the self, the two overlap in time; redefining the relationship begins before redefining the self is completed. Both these processes provide new biographical trajectories for caregivers and care recipients individually and together as a dyad. The development of new life patterns is life recreated.

According to Chesla et al. (1994), relationship issues are paramount to family members in their everyday lives, and qualitatively distinct forms of relations between ill members and other family members are evident. One member in the relationship is assumed to be the passive recipient of care, holding less interpersonal power yet imposing demands and burdens. In a parallel way, the caregiving member is assumed to be an active provider, possessing relatively greater interpersonal power but at risk of negative outcomes, because of the burdens and strains experienced. Chesla et al.'s work on caregiver–care receiver relationships in the context of AD showed three categories of responses: continuous, discontinuous, and continuous yet transformed. Despite the changes in the patient, family members belonging to the continuous group continued to define themselves in relation to the patients in ways that parallelled their relations prior to the disease. Another group of family members who saw their relationship as discontinuous described the AD patient as fairly lost to them, but remained committed. These family members found ways to relate to the patient as the symptoms progressed and continued to adapt ways of relating as the AD person's capacities became more restricted. In the continuous but transformed relationship, family members saw the patient's behaviour as having been present earlier but interpreted it in new ways.

Blieszner and Shifflett (1990) detail the relationship changes over time between spouses and between parents and children in the context of a family member with AD. Respondents recalled the relationship prior to symptom onset where companionship and shared activities were enjoyed and family roles and responsibilities were distributed. When symptoms appeared but were not diagnosed, changes in the patients' behaviour could not be explained and various possibilities such as tumours, hearing loss, personality changes and old age, were explored. Knowledge of the diagnosis brought both sadness and relief. Respondents were more patient and accepting of their loved ones' behaviour once they knew the reason. Six months after the diagnosis, affection remained fairly stable despite the lack of reciprocity and companionship and the role reversals. Caregivers' growing dissatisfaction with the relationship did not preclude the provision of care. A year later, respondents stated that their relationship had changed from being close and personal to being that of a caregiver. The need for closure was expressed. Overall, the situation of nonvoluntary relationship decline results in a loss of personal control with no special markers to ease the transition.

In a small grounded theory study of family members who cared for the AD family member, Orona (1990) focused on the identity loss of the AD patient and its impact on the dyadic relationship over time. Using a social constructionist framework, Orona noticed that temporality was an important subjective aspect of the caregiving experience. Facets of the temporal experience were the use of memories to maintain the identity of the AD person, the re-enactment of meaningful social interactions with the AD person, and the use of memories as a basis for constructing new images for the future. Caregivers were found to engage in identity maintenance via everyday activities with the AD family member, and when reciprocity was lost, these relatives worked both sides of the relationship or took on both the caregiver's and AD patient's social roles in order to continue some part of the past interactions.

In her grounded theory study, Hirschfeld (1993) developed a concept of mutuality in caregiver–care receiver relations. Mutuality was defined as the caregiver's capacity to find gratification in the relationship with the impaired person, positive meaning from the caregiving situation, and a sense of reciprocity even in situations where the elder care receiver had severe dementia. Most striking was Hirschfeld's finding that the higher the mutuality in the relationship, the less likely the caregiver was to consider institutionalisation of the elder.

Chesla (1991) illustrates the interface between caregiver–care receiver interaction and the provision of care through four categories. In engaged care, parents continued to care for their offspring and to show an understanding and acceptance of their sometimes difficult and inappropriate behaviours. In conflicted care, parents showed little understanding or acceptance of their offspring's illness and behaviour and tried to minimise any impact on their own lives. Even though these parents continued to provide care, their approach often resulted in conflict and extreme dissatisfaction with their life situation. In managed care, parents were characterised as being active and objective in managing and learning to cope, yet they found the experience very draining and expressed a strong need for breaks from the work of caring. Finally, distanced care was evident mostly in fathers who entrusted the direct caregiving work to another member of the family, most often their wives, yet reported feeling emotionally hurt and excluded from their son's or daughter's lives.

Midlarsky (1994) believes that when the caregiver is motivated by genuinely selfless, other-oriented and empathic nurturance, both he/she and the care recipient benefit. Care receivers benefit because the authentic feeling behind the care facilitates psychological well-being, while caregivers report less burden because problems of inequity and relational imbalance are not experienced.

RECIPROCITY

By and large, caregiving is associated with unidirectionality and patient passivity, where support flows in a linear fashion from the caregiver to the care receiver. However, in truth, the care receiver is an active agent of the exchange and supports the caregiver (Fergus et al. 2002). Undoubtedly, due to illness-based restrictions, the nature of support is different to that received prior to the illness, but it continues to be provided and its value for the caregiver and the care receiver cannot be undermined (ibid). This reciprocity has received limited attention in the literature (ibid.; Walker et al. 1992).

Neufeld and Harrison (1995) investigated reciprocity as a dimension of social support for women caring for cognitively impaired elders and mothers caring for premature infants. Using three to four open-ended interviews with 40 caregivers and significant others over an 18-month period, they identified reciprocity variation: reciprocity (give and take, balancing), generalised reciprocity (giving to others), constructed reciprocity (observing a care recipient for response), and waived reciprocity (no expectation of reciprocity due to the incapacity of the ill person). Reciprocity was demonstrated by women who kept a mental list of people who had assisted them. Generalised reciprocity was illustrated by those who gave without expectation of benefit. Constructed reciprocity was significant to the quality of the caregiver–care recipient relationship, and caregivers looked for cues indicating that the care recipient had benefited. Caregivers who built constructed reciprocity experienced a positive affect, increased self-esteem, and greater satisfaction from caregiving.

Fergus et al. (2002) conceptualised patient-provided support for spouse caregivers in the context of prostate cancer as 'active consideration', which captured patients' inclinations to expand their perspective to include that of their partners as well as patients' purposive attempts to buffer the impact of the illness on their partners. Active consideration comprised four domains of easing spousal burden, keeping us up, maintaining connectivity and considering spouse. Easing spousal burden implied diminished demands placed on the caregiver including minimising inconvenience, contributing to managing the household, protecting from fear and frustration, and working towards a speedy recovery. Keeping us up prevented the patient and partner from preoccupation with negative feelings through the balancing of mood and the adoption of a positive attitude. Considering spouse expanded patients' self-focus to include consideration of spousal perspective and needs by recognising the impact on the partner, seeing the spouse's perspective, exhibiting thoughtfulness and sensitivity, and encouraging spousal independence. Maintaining connectivity promoted experiences of bonding between partners at each stage of the illness by means of sharing feelings, spending time together and expressing affection. Overall, the nature of the support was predominantly emotional since functional limitations precluded concrete assistance. Nonetheless, positive feelings in both caregivers and care receivers and a strengthening of their relationship were reported, along with lower levels of burden and greater motivation to provide care in the caregiver.

Care receivers who see themselves as active participants in the relationship should have positive self feelings as well as positive social interactions. Douglass (1997) examined the relationship between reciprocal support and psychological adjustment of cancer patients and their spouses. She found that both patients and spouses reported less depression and higher self-esteem when exchanges of support were perceived to be balanced and high.

Similarly, when caregivers perceive recipients to be making a contribution in return for the care received, they may be able to focus on the positive aspects of their relationship with the receivers. Walker et al.'s (1992) exploratory study of the perceptions of the aid given to caregiving daughters by their care receiving mothers in return for the daughters' help found that a majority of both mothers and daughters perceived the mothers as giving aid to the daughters in return for the help received. The type of aid most commonly perceived was love. The mothers also gave information or advice while half of them reported giving money. A majority of daughters who received aid from their mothers described that aid as invaluable. The study supports the view that care receiving mothers are actively engaged in relational exchanges with their caregiving daughters, and that reciprocity is valued in the caregiving relationship.

Ingersoll-Dayton et al. (2001) examined the help received from ageing care receiving parents by sandwiched-generation caregiving couples who were also employed (couples who care for both children and ageing parents). Their findings extended Bengston and Roberts' (1991) functional solidarity framework by suggesting that such help is a mixed blessing. That is, receiving emotional support is beneficial in terms of the quality of relationships and improved self-ratings of caregiving performance. However, financial assistance, child care and household-related help were problematic since respondents worked less effectively at paid employment because of caregiving concerns. Moreover, negative emotions were precipitated by the help because respondents felt guilt about being dependent, annoyance over unsolicited help and frustration when assistance was inadequate.

SYSTEMATISING THE FIELD

As research on family caregiving gets underway, providing rich insights into a multifaceted and complex concept, attempts to systematise the substantive area through the development of models and paradigms have been made.

Given and Given's (1994) integrative model (linking continuing care across formal and family care systems) depicts the interplay between formal and informal systems. The formal system
has been separated into acute and continuing care, and system
decisions are influenced by patient age and comorbidity. Continuing therapy is determined by, as well as determines, the site
and stage of the illness, patient needs for symptom relief, patient
requirement for assistance with self-care, and patient ability to
perform customary activities. Family care is relevant because the
capacity of family caregivers to adequately implement complex
therapeutic regimens, to manage home-care technology, to meet
patient needs for symptom management, to help patients follow
good dietary regimens, and to maintain patient emotional health
influences patients' capacities to remain in treatment and to benefit
from it through favourable treatment outcomes. Benefits can be
maximised through the optimal interaction of formal and informal
systems of care, which is contingent on caregiver-care receiver
living arrangements, caregiver role set and the capacity of the
caregiver to incorporate added demands into his/her schedule.
The efficacy of such a model should be reflected in improved
patient and caregiver outcomes.

Young and Kahana (1994) provide a conceptual approach to
caregiver–care receiver interactions based on research with later
life chronic illness. Their dyadic outcome model describes four
possible caregiver-care receiver outcomes ranging on a continuum
from positive to intermediate to negative. The scenarios include
either both caregiver and care receiver prospering, only the
caregiver prospering and the care receiver declining, only the
care receiver prospering and the caregiver declining, or both
caregiver and care receiver declining. The first and last scenarios
represent symmetrical outcomes while the second and third situations speak of mixed outcomes.

Kazak and Christakis (1994) adopt a social ecological systems
perspective to understand how childhood chronic illness recipro-
cally impacts upon individuals and systems internal and external
to the family. This provides a framework by which contextual
factors affecting the experience of family care for chronically ill
children can be understood. The model identifies four concentric
spheres of influence such as microsystem, mesosystem, exosystem
and macrosystem. Reciprocity which emphasises the interactive,

rather than linear, nature of family care forms a cornerstone of the framework. Transitions which underscore the importance of change, both expected and unexpected, make up a critical aspect. The complex interrelatedness of the various components is underscored. Through this holistic analysis, issues that impact on caregiving and care receiving can be identified for further research and intervention.

Undoubtedly, the aforesaid models form an important contribution since they take specific findings a step further and transform them into higher order general conceptualisations. However, they are limited by their application to particular aspects of caregiving or depiction of specific groups.

Kahana et al.'s (1994) paradigm, on the other hand, comprehensively maps out the key components of caregiving in formal and informal care settings. According to them, in both these settings, caregiving includes personal and social contexts, and spatial, transactional and temporal dimensions. The personal context considers caregivers, care receivers and the caregiver–care receiver dyad in the formal and informal set-ups, whereas the social context encompasses informal groups (such as family and friends), the health service system and societal institutions (such as governments and policy-making bodies). The three dimensions address who is involved in caregiving and how this role allocation came about (spatial), what processes caregiving entails (transactional), and illness phase, life cycle and historical influences relevant to caregiving.

Kahana et al.'s (1994) contribution is clearly encompassing and inclusive, being viable across a wide range of family caregiving situations. Yet, its drawback lies in the fact that it is a mere listing of the various dimensions and does not indicate linkages or causality.

THE ROAD AHEAD

The literature presented so far gives the reader an idea of the available knowledge in the field. There is considerable work elucidating the concept of family care, the organisation of care, outcomes of caregiving for caregivers, and the caregiver–care receiver relationship. Attempts to develop models and paradigms are also being made. However, a closer look at the studies highlights a number of lacunae that need to be addressed if our understanding of the phenomenon and its complexities and subtleties is to be sharpened.

For example, research endeavours in family caregiving have essentially focused on families that do provide home care, rather than those that do not. They have focused, more specifically, on the primary caregiver, examining the kinds of care he/she provides, the motives for caregiving and the costs of caregiving. Since women provide most of the care, much of caregiving research has restricted the sampling to women caregivers. The intent of such research is to describe commonalities in the caregiving process. The result is a homogeneous portrait of caregiving provided by highly committed female individuals who are motivated by attachment and obligation. Caregiving in the context of the larger family system, permitting examination of secondary caregivers as well as of male participants, has rarely been studied (Kramer 2000; Pyke and Bengston 1996).

Not only has emotional support as an integral part of caregiving been ignored (Keefe and Fancey 2000), but care receivers are also almost completely sidelined in family caregiving inquiries (Conger and Marshall 1998).

Literature on caregiving is sketchy with respect to young caregiving families. For instance, there is limited research available on how families cope with handicapped youngsters, premature babies, children with chronic illnesses, and children with congenital problems, particularly those arising from teratogens. Another gap is the caregiving activities of older families, especially where grandparents care for ill/disabled grandchildren (Aldous 1994).

Despite the general acceptance of the notion of a caregiving career, longitudinal studies in the field remain relatively sparse. Though these studies are important to highlight the changing demands of the illness and the concomitant adjustments and costs/ benefits to caregivers and their families, as well as to demonstrate the interface between family care and formal services, especially institutionalisation (Hooyman and Gonyea 1995), most approaches are cross-sectional. There is a predominance of quantitative methods, and reviews of literature have identified a paucity of research that relates to the lived experience of home care from either the family caregiver's or care recipient's perspective (Conger and Marshall 1998).

It need not be further reiterated that despite the advances in the study of family care, much needs to be done, and critiques of the field so far provide the necessary direction, serving as signposts in our quest to fully uncover the complexities of the phenomenon.

In conclusion, though the family care literature essentially speaks about the care provided at home, there is evidence that suggests that family care operates even when the care receiver is institutionalised. Institutionalisation is thought to enable a transition of caregiving responsibility and burden from the informal to the formal system of care. A growing body of research, however, suggests that responsibilities of family members continue after an elderly member has been admitted to a long-term care (LTC) facility, but perhaps in an altered way (Fancey and Keefe 1994). Family members regularly visit institutionalised relatives, during which time they perform instrumental and recreational care tasks, provide emotional support and maintain the relationship (Keefe and Fancey 1997; Ross et al. 1997). 'Preservative caregiving', which includes taking residents on day trips, placing memorabilia in the resident's room and teaching staff about the uniqueness of the resident and his/her preferences, is also undertaken (Bowers 1988). Family members report that their indirect responsibilities (i.e., manager, not provider of care) increase following institutionalisation, while direct responsibilities (i.e., actual performance of caregiving activities) are limited. Indirect responsibilities include playing advocacy roles, overseeing the quality of care provided, being on call and maintaining a relationship with the staff. Direct responsibilities involve providing emotional support and, if required, physical support, providing personal comfort and being a link to the community. In addition to specific tasks with their elderly relative, family members also become engaged in administration, advocacy, and activities for all residents (Keefe and Fancey 2000). The literature thus reinforces the centrality of the family in caring for its members, regardless of their place of residence, and disputes the myth that family members abandon their relatives following admission to an LTC facility (Fancey and Keefe 1994). On the contrary, most family members indicate no change in their perceived responsibilities towards their family member in the post-institutionalisation phase (Keefe and Fancey 2000).

Predictions are being made about an accelerating sandwich-generation caregiving population. Here, substantial numbers of middle-aged caregivers with chronically ill adult children will also have to cope with caregiving for aged parents. Unless there are viable supplemental/alternative resources, caregivers will undergo severe role strain that will damage their physical health and cause emotional distress (Lefley 1996).

2
HIV/AIDS AND FAMILY CARE

The advent of HIV and AIDS is not seen simply as the appearance of a new disease that could be easily integrated into an existing order of things. It is perceived as a rupture of society (Duttmann 1996). From an infection that at first was seen as affecting gay men in a few American cities, it has grown into a pandemic. Nelkin et al. (1990: 1) maintain that AIDS 'is no ordinary epidemic. More than a devastating disease, it is freighted with profound social and cultural meaning. More than a passing tragedy, it will have long-term, broad-ranging effects on personal relationships, social institutions and cultural configurations ... the effects of the epidemic extend far beyond their medical and economic costs to shape the very ways we organize our individual and collective lives'.

AIDS represents the emergence of a metaphorical illness and the discovery of a perfidious virus. It jeopardises scientific research and social norms and institutions. It reveals, catalyses and increases the flaws and gaps between the rich and the poor and between the north and the south, bringing to the fore social fissures. It awakens long-forgotten intolerant discourses and recalls ancient fears. It emphasises technological advances (Paicheler 1992). It prompts the most brave and generous acts, yet provokes the most mean-spirited and non-rational behaviour (Teguis and Ahmed 1992). For Western nations which no longer experience big epidemics, AIDS has put an end to their peace of mind (Paicheler 1992).

AIDS has brought about a general awareness of a new situation where the risk of illness is constantly present. People must learn to live with this risk and are likely to become more conscious of it as progress is made in predictive medicine. Although social science has not paid much attention to the 'risk of illness' situation, AIDS research has focused on temporality, uncertainty, risk-management and body control. This helps to understand what it means to have a positive status. To be HIV-positive is to learn that you are carrying a transmissible, lethal virus. Even though you may not be already sick, you are dangerous to yourself and to others, and you know neither when nor how you will fall ill. As a result, certain risks must be managed in a situation of uncertainty (Pierret 2000).

The shadow of stigma is never far from HIV/AIDS, arising from its initial associations with 'risk groups', from its sexual mode of transmission, from its contagious nature and from its fatal consequences (Cargan and Ballantine 2000). Stigma has brought to light numerous complex issues, such as the importance of confidentiality, the management and consequences of secrecy, the biases within society and within the health profession, the limits on positive people's expectations of care and support and the pain of experiencing discrimination. The result of perceiving AIDS as the adversary is to consider positive people as casualties and victims, exacerbating a sense of hopelessness and impotency. Victims are placed on a continuum of 'innocence' or 'guilt', which determines their worthiness of our compassion, and of deservedness or nondeservedness of the disease (Teguis and Ahmed 1992).

It is an indisputable fact that dealing with a disease such as HIV/AIDS constitutes an enormous challenge, which can be met only through a broad interdisciplinary approach that spans prevention, treatment, care and rehabilitation. Particularly in the absence of a biomedical solution, it becomes the mandate of social scientists to deliver ever-increasing contributions for the adequate conception and assessment of prevention and care (Pollak 1992).

The Joint United Nations Programme on HIV/AIDS (UNAIDS) (2002) estimates 40 million people worldwide to be living with the HIV virus. In India, the first HIV case was reported in a female commercial sex worker (CSW) in Madras in 1986 (National AIDS Control Organisation/NACO 2001a). In 2001, NACO estimated 3.97 million HIV infections, 3.31 million of which were in the 15–49 age group. The data further point out that Maharashtra, Tamil Nadu, Andhra Pradesh, Karnataka and Manipur have the highest rates, whereas Arunachal Pradesh, Assam, Meghalaya, Sikkim and Rajasthan report little or no seropositivity. Similarly, urban areas have higher rates than rural areas, while the number of male cases outweighs that of females (NACO 2001a). Micro-level studies add to these data by pointing out the growing incidence of seropositivity among rural populations; married, monogamous women; housewives; voluntary blood donors; women attending antenatal clinics; and paediatric HIV/AIDS cases (see, for example, Gangakhedkar et al. 1997; Solomon et al. 1998; Verma and Roy 2002). The spread of the HIV infection in India is mostly driven by heterosexual transmission (Panda 2002). A majority of women have no risk factor other than being married to their husbands and increased HIV infections in young women in the reproductive age group is accompanied by an increase in vertical transmission and paediatric AIDS (Verma and Roy 2002). Thus, though the epidemic was initially viewed as being primarily concentrated among people practising high risk behaviours, it has now become quite clear that it has spread to several sub-groups of the general population that do not display high risk behaviour (NACO 2001b; Panda 2002; Verma and Roy 2002). It is believed that if current transmission rates continue, India will soon have the largest concentration of AIDS-affected individuals in the world (Verma and Roy 2002).

The numerous predisposing and precipitating risk factors that either directly or indirectly facilitate HIV transmission in India are intricately linked with social and cultural aspects of life, including migratory patterns, increasing urbanisation, poverty, illiteracy, subordinate status of women, high rates of sexually transmitted diseases (STDs) and intravenous drug use and the widespread prevalence of unsafe sexual practices. Inadequate access to health information and services are found to affect the ability of the population, particularly those at risk (including women), to protect themselves (see Verma and Roy 2002, for a detailed discussion).

The majority of HIV/AIDS-related services in India centre around primary prevention, and are provided mainly by the public and to some extent the voluntary health sectors. Yet, these are inadequate in content, volume and orientation, and leave much to be desired in terms of their effectiveness. They, therefore, have done little to stymie the growth of the infection (Aggarwal et al. 1997; Asthana 1996; Gupta and Panda 2002; Panda 2002; Rawat 1999; Ramasubban 1998; Sathiamoorthy and Solomon 1997; Sethi 2002; Thomas et al. 1997; Verma et al. 1999).

Treatment and support do not occupy centre stage. The former is provided by the public and voluntary sectors, and to a lesser extent, by the private sector. Support, on the other hand, is almost exclusively the domain of the voluntary sector, though given the disproportionate ratio of the number of people in need of support versus the amount of support available, many receive insufficient or no support at all (Aggarwal et al. 1997; Asthana 1996; D'Cruz 2003a; Gupta and Panda 2002; Rawat 1999; Ramasubban 1998; Sathiamoorthy and Solomon 1997; Sethi 2002; Thomas et al. 1997; Verma et al. 1999).

Ultimately, the grossly inadequate development of secondary and tertiary health interventions burdens the population with the responsibility of providing home-based healthcare for ill family members. In other words, families have to undertake the caregiving role and bear the cost of the care for their sick members. This development is in keeping with the dictates of structural adjustment which advocates cutbacks in social sector expenditure and policies of community care (Duggal 1995; Qadeer 2000; Tulsidhar 1993), even though it is a well-known fact that community care is a mere euphemism for family care (McCann and Wadsworth 1994). Further, such practices are aligned with global policies on HIV/AIDS intervention, which promote the continuum of care model as the internationally recognised and recommended ideal form of secondary and tertiary prevention to deal with the infection (see Global Programme on AIDS/GPA 1995).

Yet, family care in HIV/AIDS poses a unique challenge because of the distinguishing features of the infection. Given the nature of the disease, it is not unlikely that the caregiver as well as the care recipient and perhaps other family members, are unwell too (Lesar and Maldonado 1997; McCann and Wadsworth 1994; Millon et al. 1989; Reidy et al. 1994; Seeley et al. 1994). Not only do caregivers have a dual role, simultaneously being clients with psychosocial needs and service providers in need of advice and information to manage ongoing care (Sosnowitz and Kovacs 1992), but they also experience extra demands, with limits on the care they can provide, alternating between periods of providing care and needing it. Further, since the pandemic has struck mainly young adults, caregiving engenders role reversals that represent major upheavals for families. Elderly parents and dependent, young children often end up performing the caregiving role, sometimes unsuited to their age. The caregiving experience in HIV/AIDS is therefore a complex one, singularly different from that of other chronic conditions (Lesar and Maldonado 1997; McCann and Wadsworth 1994; Reidy et al. 1994). The role of the family in the provision of care in HIV/AIDS is considered to be much more stressful than it is in other diseases. With the virus targeting mainly young adults in the sexually active and economically productive age group, with its stigmatising and terminal nature, and with the prolonged 'living-dying interval' (Pattison in Stephenson 1985: 80), the challenges of caregiving in HIV/AIDS have become a much discussed issue. Yet, in terms of empirical investigations, family care remains one of the least studied areas. The essential foci of existing studies, as we shall see in the following sections, have been on various categories of caregivers, on factors that impinge on the provision of care, and on caregiver outcomes. Insights are thus limited, with many gaps left to be examined. Within this, Indian literature on HIV/AIDS and family care is markedly limited. The sections which follow, therefore, largely rely on Western and African literature.

CAREGIVERS OF SEROPOSITIVE PEOPLE

The organisation of family care in HIV/AIDS presents a complex picture, reflecting the expanding conceptualisation of the family that has gained visibility as a result of the pandemic (Heaphy et al. 1999; Levine 1994). Due to familial arrangements of people living with HIV/AIDS that extend beyond blood, marital and legal ties to include self-determined bonds, caregiving within the family is not necessarily feminised. Thus, besides wives, mothers, sisters, sisters-in-law, daughters and grandmothers being caregivers (Ankrah 1994; Barlow 1994; Bharat 1996; Campbell 1999; D'Cruz 2003a; Grunseit and Kippax 1992; Reidy et al. 1994; Seeley et al. 1994; Singhanetra-Renard et al. 1996; Wilson 1994; UNAIDS 2000), there are instances of males such as lovers, friends and buddies performing this role (Brennan and Moore 1994; McCann and Wadsworth 1994). Moreover, in contrast to the conventional notion of the elderly being cared for by their adult offspring, in HIV/AIDS, there are instances of aged parents caring for their adult children and grandchildren (Ankrah 1994; Poindexter and Linsk 1998, 1999). Child caregivers are not uncommon either (UNAIDS 2000, 2001a). All these people constitute a precious resource (UNAIDS 2000).

WOMEN AS CAREGIVERS

Notwithstanding the changing definition of family and its impli-cations for the organisation of care in the context of HIV/AIDS (Heaphy et al. 1999; Levine 1994), in developing countries, fam-ily caregivers in HIV/AIDS are mainly women (Ankrah 1994; Barlow 1994; Bharat 1996; Bharat and Aggleton 1999; Campbell 1999; D'Cruz 2003a; Grunseit and Kippax 1992; Seeley et al. 1994; Singhanetra-Renard et al. 1996; Wilson 1994). As society's tradi-tional caregivers, women carry the main psychosocial and physi-cal burdens of AIDS care, even though they have the least control over, and access to, the resources they need to cope effectively (de Bruyn et al. 1995). Invisible care by women is already a fea-ture of life in communities profoundly affected by HIV. In their experience of providing care, women may feel pain and anger after finding out the sexual orientation or lifestyle of their partner or child. Caring for HIV-positive children is very distressing and mothers experience unvoiced pain when they become sounding boards for their child's anger and frustration. Emotional strain relating to uncertainty, isolation, lack of support, fear of infection, implications of the diagnosis and impending death, is common. Not only does caregiving involve arduous work, but women may also have to take up paid employment, often outside the house, to provide financially for the members of the family after the earner loses his job or earning capacity. On the other hand, a woman may be pressurised into giving up paid employment in order to care for an infected family member at a time when money is badly needed in the HH. The cost and availability of healthcare adds to her burden in a situation where she faces discrimination due to her association with HIV/AIDS. Women, thus, have to deal with multiple demanding roles, which bring on tremendous strain and they cope, being the mainstay of families already disadvan-taged by poverty and deprivation and of families whose lives may be characterised by poor housing, poor educational opportunities, difficult family relationships and chemical dependence. Seen as being able to cope, they are rarely asked about what help and support they need to be able to do the job of caring. Their own needs are the least well met, if at all. That is, not only do they put their needs last, but society also does not pay much attention to their needs (Ankrah 1994; Barlow 1994; Bharat 1996; Campbell 1999; D'Cruz 2003a; de Bruyn et al. 1995; Grunseit and Kippax 1992; Huby et al. 1993; Mane 1995; Wilson 1994).

The situation is further complicated when women caregivers are seropositive and in need of care. By and large, such women have to continue with their caregiving role. Women living with HIV in the community usually bear the responsibility for child care, housekeeping, earning, health and social work department appointments, and their own illness, as well that of their partner, their children and other family members. Thus, they have no one to either take over their responsibilities or to provide them with care. Moreover, given the extent of responsibility on them, their attention is channelised towards fulfilling these responsibilities and hence they tend to neglect their own needs until it is no longer possible to overlook them (Ankrah 1994; Barlow 1994; Bharat 1996; Campbell 1999; D'Cruz 2003a; de Bruyn et al. 1995; Grunseit and Kippax 1992; Huby et al. 1993; Mane 1995; Wilson 1994).

Hackl et al. (1997) documented HIV-positive women caregivers' experiences in their study. They found the primary concerns of such women centred around stigma, child concerns and caretaking roles, social support needs, concerns about death, dying and despair and HIV/AIDS information needs. Women feared disclosing their HIV status because of perceived family, peer and societal rejection. They opined that it would be better to suffer in silence than to face social judgements and described difficulties in establishing and maintaining intimate relationships. Parental caregiving issues were the second most frequently raised concern of these HIV-infected women. Other concerns frequently involved identification and quality of guardianship. They were also worried about the inability to protect their children from crises and about stigma resulting from the parent's diagnosis. The women's responses indicated two significant areas of social support concern: a strong desire for support networks and a fear of reaching out because of the ostracism that can follow HIV status disclosure. Perceived feelings of isolation were consistently present throughout these women's interviews. The primary reason given by the women for wanting social support was to have an environment in which they could openly share their fears and feelings with people who were experiencing the same types of isolation and pressure. Intense feelings of hopelessness, fear of suffering during the dying process and suicidal thoughts were consistently discussed by these participants. The belief that the HIV diagnosis meant imminent death and the perceived lack of psychosocial resource supports were reported as key information issues. The lack of medical information regarding the prognosis for living with HIV created confusion for many of these women. The women knew they had HIV, but most felt that they knew little else about the disease. Even after diagnosis, several women did not understand transmission routes, how to get HIV prevention information, or how to find physicians who specialise in HIV/AIDS treatment. Most women interviewed believed that an HIV diagnosis meant that they had AIDS and would die within a year or two. Several had had thoughts of suicide immediately after being diagnosed (Hackl et al. 1997).

A theme that emerged in the interviews was the women's ongoing struggle to balance their own health concerns with the demands and needs of their families. Silence regarding the HIV diagnosis required hiding medication, or as in the case of one woman, refusing medication to avoid children's questions about their health. Medical appointments were often scheduled when children were in school or when child care could be arranged. Even women who cared for dying partners rarely told their children of their own need for hospitalisation. The women reported that increased HIV-related fatigue was handled by sleeping during the day when possible. However, this resulted in increased guilt when HH chores and meal preparations were not completed by the time children arrived home from school. All the women described strong feelings of guilt and concern for their children's future. Regardless of the transmission route, the women generally expressed guilt about becoming infected. Several women perceived that becoming infected meant that they had failed their children. Although two of the women had disclosed their HIV illness to older children, most mothers were reluctant to disclose the illness until it was absolutely necessary. The tenor of these women's interviews indicated their need to maintain a sense of parental status and dignity and to protect their children's well-being (Hackl et al. 1997). The emotional strain of the experience was, therefore, overwhelming.

When women reach a stage in the infection where they need care, parents, siblings, older children or outside caregivers may step in as primary caregivers, changing the family organisation. Yet, such role reversals, where from being a caregiver and a protector, the woman is now in need of care and is a potential source of infection and family disruption, were found to upset the women greatly. Anticipating such a role reversal and its implications was a major reason why some women were earlier reluctant to inform the family of their seropositive status and of their needs, allowing themselves to undergo considerable stress and loneliness (Miller and Goldman 1993).

PARENTAL CAREGIVERS

Parents caring for an adult child with HIV face multiple challenges. Besides the loss of aspirations, the infection represents a life-cycle shift for them. At a time when parents may have already completed the task of or may have been in the process of launching their children and considering some of their major life tasks over, the presence of the infection and the caregiving it engenders dictate that they undergo a role reversal. They experience a disruption in the natural order of families, resuming a long discarded role as guardian or decision maker for their child. They also go through the pain of having to watch their offspring die and of having to outlive their child. Instead of the usual family developmental tasks at this phase, that is, personal identity development among members, the key developmental tasks becomes renewing and revising the cohesion issues of bonding and attachment. Adaptability may also be taxed in cases of homosexual or intravenous drug user (IVDU) seropositives where parental caregivers experience the added stressor of the initial acknowledgement of homosexuality or drug abuse of their adult child. Instead of being able to count on their adult children in their old age, they have to care for them and sometimes for their children too. Depending on their class, this may be with little or no financial support. Physical strength and capability may also be waning, while the existence of some physical ailment in the parent cannot be overlooked (Brennan and Moore 1994; Sewpaul and Mahlalela 1998; Wiener et al. 1994).

In a study of parental caregivers of HIV-infected adult offspring in Thailand, older parents were seen as being greatly motivated and dedicated to improve the well-being of their children and acted as major caregivers. They were intimately involved in all facets of their child's experience. The inquiry showed that routine caregiving required extensive time, and is augmented during the final stages of the infection when the positive person needs help with basic bodily functions. Financial demands can accumulate till a point where the child's and parent's resources are exhausted. Parents solicit help from other relatives for caregiving with varying degrees of success, paying expenses and providing emotional support. In addition, viewing their role in terminal stage caregiving as part of the responsibility that parents have for their children (regardless of age), refusing to view their child as a burden and avoiding blame for their son/daughter's infection, all help the Thai parents to cope. Social stigma and the fear of it are not as extreme in Thailand as in other countries, but it does inhibit some parents from moving beyond the family for assistance, including approaching formal sources. Nonetheless, parents display strong wills to help their children as much as possible. Sometimes, in desperation, they seek treatment from traditional healers, at high costs. Despite serving as a link between the healthcare system and the community at large, the needs of parental caregivers were found to be largely overlooked (UNAIDS 2001b).

In many but not all paediatric HIV cases, a parent serves as the informal caregiver. The child who is HIV-positive, in his/her need for normal human nurturing, becomes doubly dependent and the natural caregiver becomes doubly burdened. The very nature of the disease, its cause and transmission and the particular relationship between the sick child and his/her natural caregiver, necessarily make the problems of AIDS different from that of other chronic childhood illnesses. The presence of the virus in the offspring represents a loss of aspirations that were nurtured by the parents. With the exception of cases of haemophilia and transfusion-related disorders in children, the presence of an infected child in the family almost necessarily means the presence of one or more infected adults, one of whom is almost always the mother. It is difficult for such a mother to provide care when she herself is frightened of being sick or is already sick and facing frequent hospitalisation. Moreover, she is riddled with guilt if she has passed on the infection to her child. The situation is worsened by the conspiracy of silence in the face of a positive diagnosis and by the social isolation attendant on maintaining such a silence. In instances of haemophilia and thalassemia, HIV adds on to an existing chronic illness, whereas in cases where the parent is negative, there is the pain of having to watch one's offspring die and of having to outlive one's child. As the burden of care becomes heavier, anxiety for the future increases and intrafamilial conflicts are heightened. The family closes in on itself, deprived of most sources of information and external support and aid. When family organisations tend to become nuclear with a poor support system, those close to them are called upon to contribute to the care of infected family members and to form a new family structure. Paediatric AIDS, with the likely infection of mother and child, evinces further loss of autonomy and increase in financial dependence. If the mother is the primary wage earner, she faces a loss of income for the time taken from work for treatment or diagnosis; if, in addition, she herself is infected, she faces the eventual loss of employment and the need for financial assistance in the form of welfare. With time, her own demands and those of her child will increase as her human and financial resources decrease. Her feelings of worth are further threatened as she is forced to relinquish the care of the child to another member. If this role is assumed by the grandmother or aunt, conflicts in the family may reintensify, as the latter assumes more or less willingly the double burden of care. Her needs are similar to, and no more likely to be met than, those of the mother (Brennan and Moore 1994; Lesar and Maldonado 1997; Reidy et al. 1994; Sewpaul and Mahlalela 1998).

Brouwer et al. (2000) observed that parental caregivers need to accept their child's seropositive diagnosis in order to be motivated to comply with the advice of healthcare workers and to provide appropriate care. However, this in turn depends on their emotional condition. Greater despair and depression interfere with compliance and health seeking. The terminal prognosis interferes with caregiving in two ways. Some parents feel no need to care since it would make no difference at all, while others report great anxiety during illness episodes, interpreting them as impending death. Parental anxieties over caregiving include poverty and the inability to purchase nutritious food and medicines.

Campbell (1999) reports that despite the strain, mothers derive a sense of purpose from caring for their HIV-positive child, though the death becomes very painful as it disrupts the natural life process in which parents are supposed to die before their offspring.

Wiener et al. (1994) found little difference in biological parents' responses between HIV-infected parents and non-infected parents, indicating that regardless of their own HIV status, these caretakers were parents first. Non-infected parents may experience more anticipatory grief, because they must accept the idea of surviving their child and of living without the child. Infected parents may experience greater anxiety due to the fear that their own health will deteriorate before that of their child. These parents must make provision for someone to care for their child when they no longer can. Brouwer et al. (2000) support this by stating that where parents themselves are seropositive, they worry about their own health and about their children's future (especially that of the infected child) after their deaths. They may try to save some money and explore extended family care, but are always haunted by the thought that no one will look after their children as they do either because of financial reasons or lack of bonding. They grieve about losing a shared future with their children and are burdened by the knowledge that they are leaving the children orphaned (Campbell 1999). According to Lesar and Maldonado (1997), if no other family member is available, foster or group home placement is required. It is estimated that 20–40 per cent of HIV-infected children now require foster or group home placement, often because birth families are too overwhelmed by their illness and lack the ability or resources to continue providing care for them.

CHILD CAREGIVERS

Children are the least acknowledged caregivers within the home. When one parent dies in a nuclear family, there is usually no one to look after the other parent and siblings (some of whom may be infected) and in these cases, children assume adult roles (D'Cruz 2001; UNAIDS 2000, 2001a; UNAIDS/UNICEF/USAID 2002). This is a version of skip-generation parenting, which involves parentification of youth (Campbell 1999). No one knows how many children act as primary caregivers, but they are believed to constitute a significant number (UNAIDS 2000). HIV/AIDS is increasingly challenging dominant conceptualisations of childhood, particularly the notion of children as dependent, passive and non-productive. This is so because the presence of child caregivers in HIV/

AIDS has brought to the fore the often overlooked contributions of children to family life and to the domestic economy. This is despite the historical presence of little mothers that have enabled many marginalised households to get by when parents were ill or working long hours. Similarly, contemporary children facing an illness like HIV/AIDS use such strategies either consciously or by default, as the most appropriate person left. The role of child caregivers conflicts with the state of childhood, prompting policy makers to state unequivocally that child caregivers should be treated as children first and as caregivers second (Chinouya-Mudari and O'Brien 1999). In their study of African migrant children living in London looking after seropositive parents, Chinouya-Mudari and O'Brien have shown that children perform a wide range of duties such as household tasks, child care, personal care for ill relatives, while also being a pillar of support to parents and other siblings who are going through emotional and physical turmoil as a result of HIV/AIDS. Children experience burden on account of their role, but this is augmented by the psychological stress and trauma of watching parents and siblings deteriorate and die. Sometimes, the cognitive stage of the child impedes them from differentiating the actual causes of the illness and subsequent death and hence, they may implicate themselves as influencing factors. Caring poses a threat to children in terms of their psycho-social development as a result of exclusion, isolation and interference with education. Child caregivers often miss school because they put the needs of the family above attending class. Sometimes they get late, are unable to do their homework and lose out on after-school activities, leading to poor attendance and low grades. Important dimensions of childhood such as time to play and to interact with peers, is another fall out. While this could be because of time, it is often attributed to parental concerns about confidentiality which makes them limit the number of associations children have. Children themselves may set limits on their social worlds, trying to keep the 'family secret', even if they are not fully aware of the reasons why. For children in the study, the loss of childhood was compounded by language barriers, because of which children found it difficult to express the stress that they were going through, or by cultural factors which inhibited disclosure of family circumstances to 'strangers'. The overall strain could lead to mental ill-health in children.

The impact of caregiving on the lives of children in Zimbabwe and Tanzania has been documented by UNAIDS (UNAIDS 2001a). Their report points out that children's education and social and recreational life is adversely affected by their caregiving responsibilities. When they do attend school, their minds are usually caught up with worries about their situation at home (ibid.). This is so because children in such circumstances not only provide care to seropositive parents, but may also be heads of households, taking charge of various tasks and of other siblings, in spite of the acute strain involved (D'Cruz 2001; UNAIDS/UNICEF/USAID 2002). Caregiving is conducted in an atmosphere of confusion since the children are usually not informed about the infection and hence, they are left to grapple with their own conclusions (D'Cruz 2001; UNAIDS 2001a). While children may face stigma if the parental diagnosis is known outside the family, they undergo severe psychological distress as they attempt to cope (D'Cruz 2001).

GRANDPARENT CAREGIVERS

When seropositive parents are unavailable or unable to provide care to HIV-infected or affected children, it is usually grandparents who take the responsibility (D'Cruz 2001; Forehand et al. 1999; Poindexter and Linsk 1998, 1999; Wiener et al. 1994). While grandparents are the first line of support, where they are unavailable, it is other relatives followed by siblings who take charge (Ntozi 1997a). Despite the high incidence of grandparent caregivers, research has hardly paid any attention to this group (Poindexter and Linsk 1998, 1999; Wiener et al. 1994). The available literature has two caveats. First, it speaks of the care receiving children as a category and does not always indicate the presence of infection among the children (D'Cruz 2001; Forehand et al. 1999; Brouwer et al. 2000; Poindexter and Linsk 1998, 1999; Wiener et al. 1994). Hence, differentiating between caregiving for affected children and for infected children becomes difficult. Second, the experiences of grandparent caregivers are usually clubbed together with those of other extended family members and termed as kinship care. Nonetheless, a reference to the literature could provide insights.

D'Cruz's (2001) and Campbell's (1999) reviews show that kinship caregivers play a key role in families where mothers can no longer care for their children. The kinship parent may be an older relative, an aunt/uncle or a grandparent, in which case it is referred to as 'skip-generation parenting'. Kinship families often learn of the infected person's diagnosis at the same time when they are requested to provide child care and hence, have to respond to two events at one time. This is trebled if any of the children are seropositive. In the case of grandparents, grappling with great emotional despair on observing the truncated life cycles of their offsprings and off-springs' families and worrying about their grandchildren's future, is common. A sense of loss is often reported, since HIV implies the premature death of offspring whose support was anticipated and counted upon as a safety net during old age. Anxiety over the grandchildren's future is palpable since they are expected to out-live their grandparents—while paucity of economic resources plays a role here, it is more the uncertainty about the reliability and trustworthiness of relatives who would then be taking over the care of the children.

The socioeconomic status of the kinship group usually reflects that of their infected family member. Where families are already disadvantaged, they experience further financial problems as a result of their commitment to child care. Moreover, in the case of grandparents, resources may be limited, given their life-cycle stage. Children experience deprivation as a result and if they are infected, then there are limits on treatment options.

Kinship caregivers have special support needs due to stigma, lack of resources and the burden of multiple infections in the same unit, but they often shy away from formal services for as long as they can, viewing reliance on them as a sign of inadequacy.

In the context of HIV/AIDS, the pool of available kinship care-givers is reducing. Some caregivers are stretched to capacity and hence suffer from burnout. Others may find it difficult to cope with multiple demands. There is a possibility that the physical and emotional strain cannot be continually managed, over a long period of time. The demands on caregivers are exacerbated if the children in their care are seropositive. Elderly caregivers such as grandparents have health problems of their own, which they tend to neglect in favour of their grandchildren. Quite often, grandparents see their own illness and death as an escape from an overwhelming situation, but for children, the death of their grandparents constitutes another round of loss. An additional outcome of skip-generation parenting is that because of the mothers' deaths, there will be fewer grandmothers to replace the current generation, resulting in a break in family continuity.

A point in favour of grandparent caregivers is that by and large, as compared to other relatives who may provide care reluctantly, exploit the children or deprive them of their rights and assets, grandparents usually work single-mindedly and selflessly for their grandchildren's well being.

GAY AND LESBIAN CAREGIVERS

HIV/AIDS has been a catalyst for expanding the definition of the family (Heaphy et al. 1999; Levine 1994), making non-heterosexual caring relations more visible and acknowledging that kinship goes beyond blood and legal ties and includes self-determination. Indeed, there is a belief that such relationships may be stronger than traditional families since they are based on support, respect and choice (Heaphy et al. 1999). Recognising caregivers in such family configurations is evident in Western literature. Intimate friends and lovers provide much of the care for the seropositive person, based on affiliation and bonding. Caregiving is a challenge here in the absence of legal protection given by biological families or marital dyads. Since both caregivers and care receivers share the same risk factors, there may be a greater identification which supports the relationship. Seronegative caregivers may experience guilt on account of their health status and this may motivate the provision of care (Brennan and Moore 1994).

Lovers and friends may be providing care with/without any influence from their care receiver's family of origin. This depends on whether the family of origin knows about their member's family of choice and how they react to it, if they do. Families who respond positively support the caregiving dyad, bringing cohesion to the situation. Where there is a tenuous relationship, because of the family of origin's inability to accept the positive person's sexual orientation/choice of partner/HIV status, a strategy of competition may operate, with the family of origin trying to take over the situation. Distress is compounded under the circumstances. This rift, along with the lack of legal recognition of alternative family arrangements, has implications for the caregiver. Despite his/her contribution, he/she may be sidelined in informal, but more particularly in formal, settings such as the healthcare system and the legal system, with the family of origin being accorded decision making, inheritance and other rights, against the positive person's wishes.

Wight (2000), based on an inquiry of HIV-infected gay caregivers, suggests that caregiving here is precursive, because the men were providing care that they themselves would need in the near future. Background factors that distinguish precursive caregiving from other forms include deteriorating physical health, AIDS stigma and alienation, and 'outness' about homosexuality, and these were found to be more consistent correlates of depression than the demands of care for the seropositive caregivers as compared to the seronegative gay caregivers. In the latter case, stress arising from the performance of caregiving tasks is more directly consequential to caregiver depression. Wight believes that precursiveness may influence the effects arising from the demands of care. In other words, HIV-positive caregivers may be better equipped to assist their care receivers without getting depressed because they anticipate their own need for such assistance in the future. In contrast, HIV-negative gay caregivers may be less apt to empathise with the care receiver, and may suffer emotionally as they perceive fewer tangible rewards for their actions. It therefore appears that poor health, alienation and stigma, and homosexuality compete with caregiving tasks as the source of primary stress in seropositive caregiving gays. Wight holds that while it is possible that precursive factors are so entrenched within the caregiving role that they are inescapably intertwined with the stress of care provision, reformulating what constitutes primary stress among precursive caregivers is important, so that significant events in the stress proliferation process can be identified and managed.

Powell-Cope (1995) studied gay couples experiencing AIDS. Both caregivers and care recipients described multiple losses, including the loss of health, independence, intimacy, privacy, and possibly the life of the person with AIDS, as well as the dissolution of a primary relationship. Couples viewed themselves as experiencing a major life transition, exemplified by three processes: hitting home, mutual protection, and moving on. Hitting home included awareness of realities, accelerating symptoms, being tested and receiving a diagnosis. Mutual protection described how partners related to each other in attempts to mitigate losses and retain essences such as independence and intimacy. Moving on meant accepting losses and uncertainty.

Sohier (1993) conducted a longitudinal study of 64 biological parents of gay men experiencing the final stages of AIDS. The finding indicates three family processes: gaining awareness, coping with the truth and acknowledging the dying. When families brought their children home for care or established themselves as caregivers in their sons' homes, they had to deal with physical deterioration and increasing bouts of illness. Anger, resentment, acceptance and deep sadness characterised their experience. Through caring for their dying sons, caregivers coped with their feelings by 'suffering about', 'caring' and 'valuing' their relationship with their adult child.

In the Indian context, field-based professionals report that the lack of documentation in this area is related to the disclosure patterns of gay seropositives. That is, gay seropositives tend to disclose only their serostatus and not their sexual orientation, for fear of rejection, preferring to give the impression that they have been heterosexually infected. Contingent on this decision, they receive their care and support within the context of the family of origin. As a result, there is no possibility of issues specific to their alternate sexuality operating in the caregiving and care receiving process.

VOLUNTEER CAREGIVERS

Volunteer caregivers could be either friends or neighbours who care out of a sense of love or duty, or they could be people who give their time to community service (UNAIDS 2000). Though they are the backbone of community care programmes in HIV/AIDS (ibid.), there has been very little research on their contribution (Campbell 1999).

A review of the limited literature on volunteer caregivers shows that the focus here so far is on the gay community. In the early days of the epidemic, when the virus was associated solely with gays and known as gay related immune disorder/GRID, members of the gay community mobilised against the disease, forming networks of formal and informal activists. An important legacy of those early days is a unique community social support system known as the buddy system. Buddy systems have been organised in communities throughout the United States. AIDS buddies are volunteers, frequently strangers to the positive person, whose purpose is to establish a relationship and socialise with the infected person. Buddies may help with routine HH tasks, but their primary role is to visit the infected individual, spend time together in social outings and convey a sense of interested caring. Buddies do not take the place of professional caregivers and seldom assume all the responsibilities of family caregivers. Yet their place, as social supports directly for the positive person, assumes prime importance during the long course of the illness. Buddies sometimes replace absent, unavailable or rejecting family members. In other families, they serve in a supportive role, never becoming central to the family role structure (Brennan and Moore 1994).

There is growing recognition that women, including wives, mothers, sisters, extended family members, friends, lesbians, infected women themselves and other women concerned about the issue, comprise an important part of the volunteer caregiver group for seropositive people. Women volunteers provide care and support to HIV-infected individuals either within their own informal social networks or through their association with AIDS service organisations (Campbell 1999).

DETERMINANTS OF FAMILY CARE

Empirical research has demonstrated the role played by a variety of factors in the family caregiving process in the context of HIV/AIDS. Wrubel and Folkman (1997) speak of the role of context in the provision of care, highlighting three variables, namely the relationship between the caregiver and the ill partner, the changing conditions of caregiving and the development of caregiving skills over time.

Bharat (1996) and Bharat and Aggleton (1999) highlight a spectrum of factors. According to their work, the size of the HH affected the distribution of caregiving tasks, though certain personal care tasks, like changing clothes or giving the bedpan, were performed only by the wife or mother. While extended HHs were good for primary caregivers, emotional care, for example, was better managed when shared with others, like in an extended HH or where there were external sources of support. Second, the severity of the illness increased the need for physical care and augmented HH involvement in care. Economic condition also affected caregiving. For example, those who could afford it, appointed nurses at home. Economic status affected the preference for hospital/home-based care. Even though home-based care was preferred as a means to support the infected family members, for lower-income HHs, small houses, water scarcity and common toilet facilities posed a great problem, making hospital care a relief. Nonetheless, all families, not withstanding their economic condition, attempted to provide care (particularly a proper diet as this was seen as a vital part of health management) to the best of their ability.

Hansen et al. (1998) further elucidate the role of economic factors. In their study based in Zimbabwe, the estimated costs of family care for a bed-ridden AIDS patient were between Z$ (Zimbabwean dollar) 556 and 841, over a three-month period. While this figure is high and represents a significant proportion of family resources, it underestimates the real costs and represents only what the family could afford and actually spent. This implies that due to economic constraints, infected people do not always receive the care they need. Since family care in HIV/AIDS has a substantial financial impact on the household, constrains employment opportunities, and in the case of lower-income groups, precipitates them into poverty, these economic consequences, in turn, operate as negative influences on the quality and quantity of further care.

The gender of the seropositive person influences the process of caregiving. Bharat (1996) and Bharat and Aggleton (1999) found that men qualified for care by virtue of their gender. Wives, even those who were infected, would neglect their own needs and exert themselves in order to provide care to their husbands. Mothers did likewise for their sons. For women, care was largely a self-managed activity. Though some women were cared for by their parents (but being conscious that they were a burden on their already poor parents, they made no demands for care), others had no one to show any special concern. In-laws were not bothered about daughters-in-law but only about their sons, often blaming the former for their sons' condition. Thus, women provided care, but were not assured of care to the same extent. In fact some women, because of their caregiving role, were allowed to stay in their in-laws' home till the husband was alive, and following his demise, were made to leave. One woman was made to leave even during the husband's lifetime in order not to tax HH resources when the husband was going to die. Women who were allowed to stay on as widows did so on terms dictated by the husband's HH, making them vulnerable. Only in one in-law HH was the wife seen as the HH's responsibility and given all care and support (Bharat 1996; Bharat and Aggleton 1999). HH involvement in care was greater for men than for women. While this differential treatment can be explained by the more advanced state of ill-health of the husband and by the socioeconomic background of the wife's parents, this is only a partial explanation. The fact remains that men do not ask for care—it is provided naturally because of their gender, whereas women have to look for it (ibid.).

The motivation to care for men came from love and duty. When the spousal relationship had been good in the past, giving care was either a matter of love and privilege, with wives feeling that they should do all that they could for the husbands, or it was a matter of love and duty, where women felt that since they had had a good life in the past with their husbands, there was no reason for them to desert their life partners now. They also felt that as Indian women, they could never leave their life partners, especially not in difficult times. Past relationships which were abusive, entailed care provided as duty with no love, but sometimes with anger and resentment. Affect is therefore a significant factor (Bharat 1996; Bharat and Aggleton 1999).

Singhanetra-Renard et al. (1996) reinforce Bharat's findings, highlighting the significance of gender, class and family type in influencing the nature and quality of care, in the context of Thailand.

D'Cruz's (2003a) work examined the experiences of a couple cohort in nuclear HHs. The study found wives to be the primary caregivers for their infected husbands but this is largely explained by the nature of family composition, stage of the family life cycle and the fact that the husbands had reached the AIDS-related complex (ARC) stage of the infection, whereas the wives were either seronegative or in the asymptomatic stage of HIV infection. Caregiving was influenced by the stage of the HIV infection, the family structure and life-cycle, the economic condition of the family, the knowledge of the terminal nature of the infection, family roles and responsibilities of the wives, and hospitalisation of the seropositive individuals. Upto the time of data collection, seropositivity in the wives in concordant couples had not hampered their caregiving ability as they were still in the asymptomatic stage. It is significant to note that with regard to the care and support given to the husband, though spousal relations may have been poor and there was anger expressed by some wives over the husbands' responsibility for acquiring the infection, care and support were never denied. It was difficult, therefore, to explain caregiving behaviour and the extent to which support came from a feeling of love versus a sense of duty. Wives appeared to be in a dilemma about this, citing love, lack of options in a nuclear HH and duty as their combined motives. One wife alluded to social pressures as well.

Ankrah (1994) points out that the employment status of the caregiver affects caregiving. While the caregiver may feel compelled to give up employment in order to provide care, the economic situation of the family may force the caregiver to combine both the roles. The long time period between diagnosis and death is also relevant since care has to be provided over the entire phase.

Seeley et al. (1994) document that lack of food, lack of money, other responsibilities, the caregiver's own health illness belief systems, stigma, presence of only children in the home making them the caregivers, fear of treatment and lack of/limited assistance from the extended family, influenced the care provided. Moreover, the presence of intervention agencies as well as the terminal nature of the illness also played a role. Millon et al. (1989) highlight the lack of preparation on the part of the caregiver and his/her other regular roles and responsibilities as relevant factors.

Surpassing this gamut of variables is one feature of the infection which makes a critical difference: the manner in which HIV/ AIDS is perceived. Of its various features, the stigmatising nature of the infection assumes primary importance in influencing how it is looked at, and this, in turn, has intense and far-reaching implications for the provision of care (Bharat 1999). Since HIV/ AIDS is associated with lifestyles that are characterised by sexual overactivity, promiscuity and permissiveness in society, such a lifestyle is attributed to the person with HIV and he/she is blamed for bringing shame upon the family. The family, therefore, may not consider it its moral duty to extend care. The family, while sheltering its HIV-positive member under its roof, may psychologically isolate the individual, leaving him/her alone for the most part of the day and/or avoiding physical care for fear of contagion. Caregivers in these families tend to perceive the disease as a deviance and the HIV-positive member as psychologically weak for giving in to sexual urges. Support and care may also be determined by the family's perception of the HIV-positive person as 'innocent' or 'guilty'. The 'guilty' are those who have brought upon the problem due to their 'uncontrolled sexual conduct', such as people with multiple partners and/or those with the power to corrupt men such as commercial sex workers (CSWs). The guilty are also those who reject the rules of society like intravenous drug users (IVDUs) and those who deny the dominant sexual order, that is, the homosexuals. Family care for such people may be less forthcoming or provided unwillingly out of a lack of choice. The 'innocent', on the other hand, may be cared for with love. These include those who have suffered infection during actions considered normal or nurturing, like those infected during blood transfusions or childbirth. Not only the family, but also the community, may come forward to help in such cases. At the same time, the perception of the 'housewife' as an 'innocent victim' of her husband's sexual conduct may not be as simple in developing societies, where the husband's family sees her as a burden and denies her care (Bharat 1995, 1999).

Songwathana and Manderson (1998) found that because people perceived HIV as dirt, danger and death, they responded to patients with considerable fear and anxiety, engendering adverse implications for the provision of care and support for the infected individual and/or his/her family. Some people maintained that infection occurred because of one's karma, and similarly, having to undertake the role of caregiver was seen as one's karma. Due to better access to AIDS information and the direct experience of seeing AIDS patients in hospitals, urban people were more likely to understand HIV transmission and risk and had more correct responses than rural people. Thus, rural people were more likely to perceive themselves to be at risk in taking care of AIDS patients than urban people. They were also less likely to provide care if their relatives and friends were infected with AIDS. Women in both urban and rural areas demonstrated considerable misinformation about the transmission of AIDS through caregiving. Rural women reported a greater precaution in contact with people who showed visible symptoms, which they regarded as indicative of high infectivity. So they were reluctant to get close to symptomatic patients and to give care and help, unless they were closely related to the patient. It is interesting that women living in areas of known AIDS cases had greater fear of contact compared to those living in areas without AIDS cases.

The stigmatising nature of the infection and the manner in which it is perceived have implications not just for patients, but impinge upon the caregivers' and families' experiences of support. Since caregiving in HIV/AIDS entails the provision of care over long periods of time, and for progressive debilitation as the infection plays out its course, caregivers undergo tremendous strain that gets exacerbated with time. Support is therefore indispensable in helping them to cope. Possible sources of this support could be friends, church members and members of a support group who are experiencing the same challenges and struggles. However, accessing support from others is often difficult for persons infected with/affected by HIV (Poindexter and Linsk 1998).

Jankowski et al. (1996), in a study of male and female confidants of seropositive individuals, reported confidants' networks to be constricted in contact and size. Confidants had diminished 'weak social ties', namely, those with acquaintances, co-workers and neighbours, and relied primarily on 'strong social ties' with family members and close friends. While limiting contacts resulted in fewer questions and a lower likelihood of having to divulge the diagnosis, using misrepresentations of the diagnosis such as maintaining a veil of pretence or a diagnostic charade, though an important means of coping, made interaction more stressful and reduced the support available. Confidants reported that having at least one person with whom they could share the truth served as a safety valve for their emotional burdens. Yet, the disclosure of diagnosis resulted in outright rejection in several cases. Moreover, where confidants provided care to HIV-infected people, the ensuing time constraints resulted in less social interaction, and hence, less support. In these various circumstances, professionals played an especially important role in providing support.

Poindexter and Linsk's (1998) work points out that caregivers of infected individuals usually received social support from persons outside the caregiving dyad and from reciprocity with the HIV-infected care recipient. In addition to these human connections, the caregivers drew support from internal and spiritual sources. External support was most often from family members and relatives, but rarely from friends. The lack of support from friends was partially due to the experience of discrimination and ostracism following disclosure of the HIV diagnosis, and partially because the respondents did not disclose their HIV caregiving to persons outside the family. Many of these caregivers manifested the need for additional social interaction and support, but felt that they could not trust anyone to receive the truth and power of their stories. The data show that this population was not likely to reach out to neighbours, friends, church members, or agencies for their emotional needs and, therefore, not likely to enjoy the stress-buffering effects of social support. That is, though they were receiving important stress-buffering effects from their families and from their faith, because they did not feel free to disclose their HIV caregiving and ask for help specific to their HIV-related needs, their choices for accessing the external support that may augment their emotional and physical functioning were limited. HIV-affected caregivers were therefore losing their community at the most trying and painful times of their lives. The consequence may be deleterious to physical and mental health, which in turn makes it more difficult to deliver care to their impaired and dying family members.

Poindexter and Linsk's other (1999) study found that because of the anticipation of HIV-related stigma, most respondents did not widely disclose the HIV-diagnosis, if at all. Consequently, they neither experienced overt HIV-related stigma nor received support that acknowledged their struggles as HIV-affected caregivers. Although most stated clearly how important church participation and spirituality were for them, respondents varied in their disclosure patterns to churches. Eleven of those who attended church had disclosed their condition to no one in their churches, including the pastor. Only two had told the pastor, two had told the pastor and a few church members, and two had gone public in their churches, but with different responses—one noticed no ramifications, and one was disappointed that none of the church members provided support. The reasons for not disclosing their condition were: HIV was a private matter; the caregiver did not feel the need for the congregation's support; or the respondent feared the implications of disclosure.

D'Cruz's (2003a) study, looking at the caregiving family's experience of support, highlights that because of the stigmatising nature of the infection, accessing support from the social circle was a difficult choice for families, even in the face of needs that could not be resolved on their own. This is in sharp contrast to both the family's earlier tradition of seeking out support from relatives and friends when the need arose, and to the process of immediately accessing support from traditional sources in the case of non-stigmatising chronic diseases such as cancer. However, once support was seen as crucial to the family's survival, the risk of inviting discrimination through disclosure did not deter them from soliciting support. It is pertinent to note that in terms of support needs, families accorded greater importance to material and financial needs, and were more likely to seek support for these rather than for emotional needs. Once they approached the social network or support system, contrary to the expectation of possible stigma, not all couples faced hostility and rejection from their social networks. There were as many families who received uninhibited support as there were those who got none or only reluctant support. Though economic position played a role among factors motivating refusal and reluctance to provide support, it was not the only important factor. The perception that the problem was an invited one that could have been averted was an important reason in one case. In another, the length of time over which support would be required, given the characteristics of the infection, was the relevant factor. Social reasons like social control and sense of duty were responsible for the provision of support in cases where assistance was reluctantly given.

While Garcia et al. (1995) and Bharat (1996) report similar findings, Bharat's study adds to this by pointing out that even when the positive person was not seen as personally responsible for the infection, the stigmatising nature of the infection hindered family members from accessing support, leaving their needs unfulfilled.

Apart from the role of the stigmatising nature of HIV infection in seeking and receiving support, caregivers report that the extended family's economic position and other responsibilities hinder their ability to assist (Ankrah 1994; Seeley et al. 1994). According to Seeley et al., the help of the extended family comes only at the time of the positive person's funeral. Though idealised by many as universal providers of limitless generosity (ibid.) and as a national strength (Ankrah 1994), the extended family's support to its members is thus questionable. Consequently, blanket statements about it being a safety net must be examined and assumptions that the extended family will be ready and able to assist sick members treated with caution. This observation is corroborated by Ntozi's (1997b) work which underscores the inadequate help that primary caregivers receive from their relatives. The reasons for this include the extended family's limited resources, other demands and stressors, a tendency to blame the positive person for the problem, an insufficient number of adults in the home, and family disputes.

CAREGIVER OUTCOMES

Family caregiving in HIV/AIDS involves five types of caregiving skills, including emotional support, hands-on care, clinical care, high-tech nursing, and healthcare advocacy. It also entails two ever-changing conditions. The first of these is the clinical course of the illness, and the other involves the shifting meanings of the clinical manifestations of HIV to both the ill person and his/her caregiver. Effective caregiving involves responding to changes in both these aspects. The changing nature of the illness means that the caregiver cannot form a rigid rule about what to do when, but has to be responsive to the process of the illness (Wrubel and Folkman 1997). Wrubel and Folkman found that the ability to deliver effective care developed over time. While caregivers underwent formal training, including courses in caregiving and training in high-tech procedures which were considered useful, it was the informal, on-the-job training that really helped them. Through the latter process, caregivers learned to distinguish those symptoms that signalled an important change in status or the reappearance of an opportunistic infection, from those that were simply part of the ongoing background of the disease. They also learned what worked in the immediate moment to ease physical or emotional distress. With experience, recurrences of infection or reappearances of a symptom no longer evoked the same level of alarm or questions about what to do that had accompanied the initial occurrence.

Caregiving for a person with HIV evokes in the caregiver a sense of vulnerability to the same illness that afflicts the care recipient, and this feeling may impinge on the care provided (Brennan and Moore 1994).

Caregivers describe caregiving as encompassing both negative and positive experiences. In Wrubel and Folkman's (1997) study, all caregivers experienced very high levels of stress. The narratives were often very explicit about the physically exhausting and emotionally draining aspects of informal caregiving. On many occasions, caregivers were interviewed when they had been working at their regular employment full time, while also staying up a good part of the night caring for their very ill partners. Their exhaustion was patent and their struggle to carry on was visible. The central stress for these caregivers was the meaning of their partners' illness, including an unexpectedly foreshortened future with the ill partner, changes in the relationship, a sense of loss of control over life circumstances, or feelings of helplessness, in the face of the partners' suffering. So, the stress of the situation was not due to caregiving, but due to what prompted caregiving. However, caregiving has a dual nature, with both positive as well as negative aspects. Narratives encompassed two core sources of positive feelings: feelings of effectiveness which are especially reinforcing when dealing with a disease that most commonly engenders feelings of helplessness, and the meaningfulness of caregiving which testified that caregiving was important and that the relationship with partners was significant and central to their lives. The co-occurrence of high levels of both positive and negative psychological states was found to be a strong, general pattern among the study's full cohort (ibid.).

The strains on those caring for seropositive people are enormous. They generally stem from financial hardship, oppressive workloads, secrecy, fear of disclosure and isolation, overinvolvement with care receivers, lack of involvement in care-related decisions, inadequate support, supervision and appreciation of their work, inadequate preparation and training for their work, lack of material resources to care, and fear of the future (UNAIDS 2000). The profound physical and emotional burden that is common to most caregivers is compounded by the stigmatising and prolonged nature of the infection, and in some cases, by their own seropositive status. While some families had no sources of social support, others who did refused to tap them for fear of stigma. Caregivers who managed on their own and who had provided care for longer periods experienced greater strain, which often made them neglect their own health and lower their guard about precautions. Positive people sometimes made unrealistic demands on caregivers, when the latter were already doing their best and were overburdened. Economically too, caregivers suffered, since they were unable to attend to their jobs resulting in loss of income, loss of job and a poor impression in the office (Bharat 1996).

Reidy et al. (1994) corroborate this. According to them, family caregivers are cognitively, socially and financially circumscribed by the impact of AIDS. They try to ignore all but the most basic and immediate of their personal needs and organise family life around the most urgent needs of the infected member. Caregivers are therefore in danger of becoming physically and emotionally burnt out—a process intensified by their isolation and the tendency to communicate only with those closest to them, a conspiracy of silence that is characteristic of AIDS (ibid.). Powell-Cope and Brown's (1992) review of studies on family caregivers in HIV/AIDS suggests that they experience significant amounts of stress, particularly in relation to isolation from families and friends due to AIDS-related stigma, and second, from uncertainty. In non-conventional families, caregivers experience considerable difficulty in coping because of conflicts between the seropositive individual and his/her family, and because of the rejection of the infected person by his/her family of origin. Ankrah (1994) reports adolescent caregivers finding their performance at school suffering due to irregular attendance, and an increasing inability to cope with school and caregiving.

Wrubel and Folkman (1997) assert that an affectionate caregiver–care receiver relationship shapes the caregiving process in a positive way. In their study, lovers and friends who provide care to HIV-positive gays, describe how their emotional connection with the care receiving person motivated them to help in any way they could. The bond between partners contributed to caregivers' capacity to sustain caregiving even under adverse conditions, and also helped them to become effective caregivers.

Caregivers experience a variety of needs. Reidy et al. (1994), using Henderson's model, studied five psychosocial needs of natural caregivers of children. General needs and within them, specific needs were identified. The need to maintain physical integrity (to understand the means of transmission of HIV, to know the ways to prevent HIV, to know how to protect the person infected by HIV from other types of infection); the need to learn (to obtain honest answers, to be informed of the evolution, prognosis and treatment of AIDS, to know how to cope with the stress associated with the condition, to learn the roles of various health professionals at the hospital, to be informed about the availability of support groups, to be consulted about who will be included in the discussion about their family problem with HIV); the need to act according to a set of beliefs and values (to discuss beliefs and values, to be respected by hospital personnel, to discuss death with professionals); the need to feel worthwhile and useful (to be supported by health professionals in maintaining their ordinary life and yet caring for the child, to have day care services made available, to maintain their social activities); the need to communicate (to be kept up to date about the child's condition, to discuss feelings, to be helped to face the reactions of those close to them, to be helped with their financial problems, to be part of a group of parents—in relation to a formal network of resource persons, to be close to a mate, to be close to the family of origin, to be close to a friend, a neighbour, or a religious group, to be able to count on those close to them—in relation to an informal group of resource persons). Other needs identified by them included the need for formal support, needs of an emotional and a functional/instrumental nature. The needs of caregivers centred around healthcare and treatment, counselling, practical and financial assistance, support, access to healthcare and medicines, employment, child care, financial assistance for medicines, food, doctors, rent and transportation, isolation and alienation, assistance with future planning, disclosure, increasing debilitation and dependence on others, emotional reactions, future of children, and shelter and legal issues (Bharat 1996; McCann and Wadsworth 1994). Bharat (1996) suggests that caregiver needs vary across income levels, with economic support being the major need for lower-income HHs.

Emotionally, caregivers undergo a myriad different feelings. Literature focuses largely on the negative, exhausting and draining ones. For instance, caregivers are known to sustain losses directly related to HIV/AIDS which are serial, multiple and cumulative in both volume and result. Each of these losses takes its toll and must be attended to. They often grieve for the people they are caring for at present as well as those who have died and who are currently ill.

Kelly and Sykes (1989) and Sosnowitz and Kovacs (1992), in describing the genesis and development of a support group for family caregivers, also document some experiences of caregivers. Kelly and Sykes listed caregiver concerns: discovery of the sero-positive status, maintenance of secrecy due to fear of stigma, loss of support, the onset of intense family conflict following disclosure, changes in family relationships following the knowledge of diagnosis, dealing with anger and hostility, coping with emotional and physical fatigue and handling the changing nature of the disease. Sosnowitz and Kovacs (1992) identified the common emotional reactions of caregivers. These include premature burial, denial, anger and depression.

It is important that caregivers' morale and well-being are protected, if the quality of care they provide and their ability to do so are to be sustained. However, though this is well recognised in principle, care for the caregiver is rarely given priority and burnout is a serious problem (UNAIDS 2000).

Besides the experiences of the primary caregivers described above, the literature also speaks about the contribution and costs of significant others. Significant others provide vital support that is of considerable benefit to the seropositive person. Cowles and Rodgers (1997) examined the experiences of this group. The basic social psychological process that dominated their lives from the time of diagnosis till the death of the HIV-infected person was of struggling to keep on top of the illness. This comprised three major aspects: accepting the challenge (coming to terms with the diagnosis and searching for information); maintaining equilibrium (closing the distance, negotiating changing relationships, normalising, hoping in the face of hopelessness); and constructing a future (planning a shared future, and anticipating death and the future without the seropositive person). Significant others in the study reported the need for support to help them through their struggle, as well as for the recognition of their relationship to and care for people living with HIV/AIDS. Overall, the findings showed that the experiences and pains of significant others are apparently not very different from those of primary caregivers, but because their contributions are generally overlooked, the trauma that they undergo is unrecognised.

A critical review of the literature on family care in HIV/AIDS presented in this chapter points out to a paucity of empirical work.

A considerable amount of the literature is based on earlier data and does not always mention any methodological and conceptual details, with empirical studies being few and far between. Many of these studies have a focus on the family in general and caregiving and support are touched upon as a part of the family experience. That is, very few have an exclusive focus on caregiving and hence, many complexities are lost. Though collectively the studies include a range of themes, respondent profiles and stages of infection, seldom does a single study encompass all these features. Moreover, despite the recognition of non-traditional family forms in the HIV/AIDS epidemic (Heaphy et al. 1999; Levine 1994), there is hardly any attention paid to unconventional families and marginalised groups, except for gay seropositive individuals and their caregivers. Within these studies, the process of care receiving and the experience of care receivers has been ignored, with the organisation of care and the caregiver–care receiver relationship receiving limited attention.

The limited understanding we have of family care in HIV/AIDS is not just an academic concern but has practical implications as well. A fragmented view hampers the creation of effective policies and programmes, underscoring the need to address the gap. Our comprehension would be greatly facilitated if the research strategy employed in empirical studies not only took care of the lacunae outlined in the preceding paragraph, but also considered the concerns of the substantive area, highlighted in Chapter 1.

3

CONTEXTUALISING THE STUDY

Qualitative research methods trace their intellectual roots to post-positivist epistemology (Schwandt 1997). Subscribing to positions such as *verstehen*, interpretive sociology, phenomenology and symbolic interactionism, post-positivists reject the imitation of the natural scientist's procedures and advocate greater attention to subjective experiences and feelings (Bryman 1988). They accept that empirical observations are important, but reject the idea that these sense experiences and reason can provide an immutable foundation for knowledge claims (Schwandt 1997). Instead, the focus is on the interpretation of social phenomena from the point of view of the meanings being employed by the people studied (Bryman and Burgess 1999). In order to do this, qualitative methods are employed since they involve an interpretive, naturalistic approach to the problem. This means that qualitative researchers study things in their natural setting, attempting to make sense of or interpret phenomena in terms of the meanings people bring to them (Denzin and Lincoln 1994) Through this process, the researcher builds a holistic and complex picture of the problematic (Creswell 1998).

Qualitative methods provide well-grounded, rich and context-ualised descriptions and explanations of experiences and process-es. They allow for the preservation of complexity and chronology, as well as the assessment of causality. Serendipitous findings and new theoretical paradigms are likely to emerge (Miles and Huberman 1994), which can be further studied and developed. Another significant purpose is to challenge the status quo and identify new paradigms or directions of inquiry (Morse 1991).

Qualitative research includes a variety of traditions, each of which is characterised by a distinct research process. By and large, these strategies have emerged from diverse disciplinary perspectives and often have sub-specialities of their own. Moreover, they are often known by different names, giving rise to a sense of confusion about the choice of approaches available. Creswell (1998), after a careful study of numerous classifications of qualitative methods, concluded that despite the varying labels, there are essentially five strategies, namely, biographies, grounded theory, phenomenology, ethnography and case studies. Table 3.1 summarises the salient features of each approach.

Qualitative methods are particularly amenable to the study of the family. This social group is characterised by unique features such as privacy, a collective consciousness not readily available to non-family members, relationships rooted in blood/marriage/adoption/self-determination and intended to be permanent, shared traditions, intense involvement and a collage of individual and group interests and experiences—in other words, families are sites of individual and shared meanings. Qualitative approaches give us windows on family processes through which we can explore patterns of interactions and negotiations of roles and relationships. They are particularly suited to study the processes by which families create and sustain their own realities, and the meanings attached to these realities. Qualitative methods also facilitate holistic studies of families where the focus is on dynamics, complexities and contexts, instead of on isolated fragments of family behaviour (Daly 1992).

RESEARCH STRATEGY

The attempt to look at the family experience of caregiving and care receiving in HIV/AIDS as a lived experience calls into play the phenomenological tradition (Creswell 1998). Phenomenology derives from the Greek word 'phenomenon' which means to show itself, to put into light or to manifest something that can become visible in itself (Heidegger in Ray 1994). According to Bishop and Scudder (1991: 5), 'phenomenology attempts to disclose the essential meaning of human endeavours'. Phenomenology includes a variety of distinctive yet related schools that are concerned with philosophy and method (Ray 1994). The two key thinkers here

Table 3.1

Dimensions for comparing five research traditions in qualitative research

Dimension	Biography	Phenomenology	Grounded theory	Ethnography	Case study
Focus	Exploring the life of an individual	Understanding the essence of experiences about a phenomenon	Developing a theory grounded in data from the field	Describing and interpreting a cultural and social group	Developing an in-depth analysis of a single case or multiple cases
Discipline origin	Anthropology, Literature, History, Psychology, Sociology	Philosophy, Sociology, Psychology	Sociology	Cultural Anthropology, Sociology	Political Science, Sociology, Evaluation, Urban Studies, other social sciences
Data collection	Primarily interviews and documents	Long interviews with upto 10 people	Interviews with 20–30 individuals to 'saturate' categories and detail a theory	Primarily observations and interviews with additional artifacts during extended time in the field (e.g., six months to a year)	Multiple sources—documents, archival records, interviews, observations, physical artifacts
Data analysis	Stories Epiphanies Historical content	Statements Meanings Meaning themes General description of the experience	Open coding Axial coding Selective coding Conditional matrix	Description Analysis Interpretation	Description Themes Assertions
Narrative form	Detailed picture of an individual's life	Description of the 'essence' of the experience	Theory or theoretical model	Description of the cultural behaviour of a group or an individual	In-depth study of a 'case' or 'cases'

Source: Creswell 1998: 65.

are Husserl and Heidegger (Cohen and Omery 1994). Husserl's eidetic-transcendental phenomenology is epistemologic and emphasises a return to reflective intuition to describe and clarify experience as it is lived and constituted into consciousness (Ray 1994). Here, it is believed that there are essential structures to any human experience and when these structures are apprehended in consciousness, they take on a meaning that is the truth of that experience for the participants. Methodologically, then, to describe the meaning of an experience from the perspective of those who have had the experience, researchers bracket their presuppositions (epoche), reflect on the experiences described and intuit or describe the essential structures of the experiences under study (Cohen and Omery 1994). Heidegger's hermeneutic-interpretive approach is ontologic, a way of being in the socio-historical world where the fundamental dimension of all human consciousness is historical and sociocultural, and is expressed through language (Ray 1994). As a research method, this approach rests on the ontological thesis that lived experience is itself essentially an interpretive process (Cohen and Omery 1994), within which presuppositions are not to be eliminated or suspended, but constitute the possibility of meaning (Ray 1994). The phenomenological task is one of explicit ontological self-interpretation (Burch 1989). It is not just watching the phenomena forming into consciousness, but an act of interpretation involving perception, whereby sense is brought from historical horizons and contextual factors to crystallise into a gestalt, whose meaning can be fully interpreted only through its history and through its relatedness to things in the world which precede, and always transcend, meaning (Langan 1970; Spiegelberg 1982).

Hermeneutic phenomenology is indisputably more ambitious than eidetic phenomenology, going beyond the meaning of what is immediately and directly manifest to our intuiting, analysing and describing, to uncover hidden meanings through the use of the ordinary and the everyday which embody clues for meanings that are usually not explicit (Cohen and Omery 1994).

Combining the goals of the Husserlian and Heideggerian schools is Dutch phenomenology, whose use in research has been vividly described by van Manen (Cohen and Omery 1994). Van Manen (1998), whose hermeneutic-phenomenological approach was adopted in the present study, portrays the methodical structure of phenomenology as a dynamic interplay between six research activities. According to him, the researcher turns to a phenomenon which seriously interests him/her and commits him/her to this abiding concern. The single mindedness of purpose results in deep introspection so that we can understand life wholly. The experience is investigated as it is lived, rather than as it is conceptualised. In other words, the attempt is to renew contact with the original experience and to focus on it as it has experienced. The researcher then reflects on the essential themes that characterise the phenomenon. A true reflection on lived experience is a thoughtful, reflective grasping of what it is that renders this experience special. The next activity is describing the experience and its essence through the art of writing and rewriting. Language and thought need to be applied to lived experience such that a precise depiction is made. In order to achieve all of this, the researcher needs to maintain a strong orientation to the fundamental question, so as to maintain direction and emerge with valid findings. He/she also needs to balance the research context by considering parts and wholes, i.e., one needs to constantly measure the overall design of the study against the significance that the parts must play in the total structure.

METHOD

In the phenomenological study, the world of lived experience is both the source and object of research. The point here is to borrow from others' experiences and their reflections on their experiences in order to arrive at a better understanding of the meaning of an aspect of human experience. Though phenomenological studies rely on traditional data collection techniques such as interviews, written responses and observations, the emphasis is not just on reporting subjective experiences of participants, but also asking what makes the phenomenon under study an essentially human one (van Manen 1998).

Following van Manen's (1998) approach, the conversational interview was used to explore and gather experiential narrative material that would serve as a resource for developing a richer and deeper understanding of the experience being studied. Interviews are preferred to protocol writing because the latter forces the person into a more reflective attitude, which may make it difficult to stay close to an experience as it is immediately lived (van Manen 1998).

Keeping in mind the difficulties of direction that emerge in unstructured interviews, the process was disciplined by focusing on the fundamental question that prompted the research, in keeping with van Manen's (1998) idea that researchers should stay as close to the experience as it is lived. That is, though the interview was unstructured, the researcher carefully considered its purpose at the outset and let this consideration shadow the process so that direction was never lost. Confusion on the part of the researcher clouds the interview, resulting in material that is either too little or too shallow or too long, irrelevant and unmanageable. Yet, the clarity of the research question did not preclude exploring issues that emerged during the interview, since the researcher was aware that they could generate important insights into the phenomenon under study.

Though such a data-gathering procedure has no scope for ready-made questions, van Manen's (1998) idea of starting with broad cues was followed. As with his observation, here too the researcher noted that these cues stimulated a process of storytelling in the participants. Since a single broad query can yield rich information on an experience, its contexts, its actors, its dynamics, nuances and consequences, its accompanying emotions and interpretations, storytelling usually proceeded without too many questions. Where responses were limited or unclear, probes were used to capture lived experience in depth and completeness. While each response was explored to the fullest, direction in the data gathering was incorporated through the use of cues.

Study Participants

As is the case in the phenomenological tradition, participants in the study should be people who have experienced the phenomenon. In this instance, the requirement was further qualified to ensure that gender, class and a range of family forms were included. Attempts were therefore made to interview male and female HIV-positive people and their caregivers, from lower, lower middle, middle and upper classes,[1] living in traditional and non-traditional families. In addition, the positive person included in the sample had to have at least one opportunistic infection. At such a stage of the infection, there is a greater likelihood of them to be in need of, and in receipt of, care. Similarly, caregivers included in the sample had to be looking after a seropositive individual in the symptomatic stage. Second, only those seropositive individuals who had shared their serostatus with their caregivers were to be included in the study, so that both caregivers and care receivers were aware of the diagnosis, and caregiving and care receiving occurred in the context of this awareness. Likewise, only those caregivers who knew their care receiver's diagnosis were to be included in the study.

Given the complexities associated with inquiries on stigmatising illnesses, difficulty in identifying and retaining participants was anticipated. The researcher, therefore, simultaneously contacted a number of organisations involved in HIV/AIDS-related work in the city of Mumbai. In keeping with ethical guidelines in HIV/AIDS research, the researcher did not approach potential participants directly. The staff of the organisation introduced the idea of, and explained the purpose of, the research to people (either seropositive individuals or their caregivers) accessing services from them, and only after they agreed and were comfortable enough, was the researcher introduced to them.

Following rapport building and soliciting their co-operation, participants signed a consent form, informing them of details of the study and of their rights if they decided to be part of the study. The location of the interview was decided by them, as also the possibility of tape-recording the interviews. At least two interview sessions per participant were desired. This would not only facilitate holistic and in-depth exploration of participants' experiences,

---

[1] Class was defined in terms of income groups. The Bombay Metropolitan Region Development Authority/BMRDA (BMRDA 1995; Draft regional plan for Bombay Metropolitan Region, 1996–2011, Mumbai, BMRDA) classification of income groups for Greater Mumbai and Mumbai Metropolitan Region was adapted and four groups identified:

(i) Lower class: Household income Rs 2,000 or less per month.
(ii) Lower-middle class: Household income Rs 2,000–6,000 per month.
(iii) Middle class: Household income Rs 6,000–12,000 per month.
(iv) Upper class: Household income Rs 12,000 and above per month.

but also allow for initial analysis and follow-up of issues emerging in the first session. The preference for two interview sessions was told to the participants during the rapport building process, in order that they could make an informed decision regarding their participation.

The process of getting participants for the study was an arduous one, largely because of the stigmatising nature of the HIV pandemic, which makes positive people and their families afraid of getting involved. Fears related to confidentiality, use of data and consequent discrimination. Time constraints due to role overload and illness severity and fluctuations were two other important considerations.

At the end of six months, despite having approached 60 potential participants, data gathering ended with 17 participants from 16 families. Of these, there were seven male care receivers, two male and three female seronegative caregivers, and five female seropositive caregivers. The age range for male participants was 26–36 years while for female participants, it was 27–60 years. While four participants belonged to the upper-income group, two belonged to the middle, three to the lower-middle and six to the lower-income group. Of these, four participants were from non-traditional family contexts, henceforth termed quasi-families. Whereas the traditional family context was defined by the presence of blood/marital ties, the quasi-family situation comprised a network of relationships that participants considered to be their families, within which care was provided (see Table 3.2).

Participants were allowed to choose the place of the interview as per their convenience. Of these, three found no problem with their homes and the interviews were conducted there comfortably. However, in the case of another three who considered their homes to be the ideal place for the interview, when the researcher went there, the curiosity of the people around made them realise that they were making themselves vulnerable to possible stigma and hence they asked the researcher to change the place of the next interview. With this change necessitating them to move out of their homes for the interview, time and role constraints impinged on the amount of time they could devote to the interview and only a single session was possible, in addition to whatever information had been collected in their homes. Though one caregiver had no objection to being interviewed in her home, time and role constraints made her consider the residential agency

Table 3.2
Sociodemographic profile of participants

Family	Gender	Age	Family income group	Seronegative caregiver/ Seropositive caregiver/ Care receiver	Family context
1	Male	34	Middle	Care receiver	Quasi-family
2	Male	28	Upper	Care receiver	Traditional
	Female	60		Seronegative caregiver	
3	Male	30	Lower-middle	Care receiver	Traditional
	Male	33		Seronegative caregiver	
4	Male	36	Upper	Care receiver	Traditional
5	Male	33	Lower	Care receiver	Quasi-family
6	Male	26	Lower	Care receiver	Quasi-family
7	Male	33	Upper	Care receiver	Traditional
8	Female	40	Middle	Seronegative caregiver	Traditional
9	Female	55	Lower	Seronegative caregiver	Quasi-family
10	Male	36	Upper	Seronegative caregiver	Traditional
11	Female	33	Lower	Seropositive caregiver	Traditional
12	Female	36	Lower-middle	Seropositive caregiver	Traditional
13	Female	38	Lower	Seropositive caregiver	Traditional
14	Female	30	Lower	Seropositive caregiver	Traditional
16	Female	27	Lower-middle	Seropositive caregiver	Traditional

(NGO C) where her HIV-positive son was admitted, to be a better option and she was interviewed there. The question of choice did not arise for five positive people living in residential facilities (NGOs B and C) and they were interviewed in the agency itself. Also, four participants preferred not to be interviewed at home (one did not get along with the family, one did not want to upset the household equilibrium, one lived in an NGO-run dormitory for street children and homeless men and one expressed a fear of publicity). A caregiver whose job involved odd working hours said that he was hardly at home and hence interviewing him in the residential agency (NGO C), where his care receiver was, was a better option, since he visited the latter there regularly.

Though the preference for at least two interview sessions was spelt out to the participants in the beginning itself, this was not possible for five participants because of time and role constraints. In these cases, the researcher explored all the relevant issues in one session itself. For participants who agreed to being, and were, interviewed twice, a preliminary analysis of the first interview was used to generate issues for clarification and further questioning in the follow-up interview, in addition to discussing emerging and unexplored areas.

A tape recorder was used in 14 cases. In these cases, once the purpose of the recorder was explained to the participants, they had no objection to its use and its presence did not appear to hinder their responses. In the rest of the cases, participants refused to allow the use of the tape recorder for fear of publicity, despite the clauses in the consent form. The researcher did not press the issue, but acceded to their wishes. Points were noted during the interviews and the conversation was written up in detail immediately afterwards.

Only individual interviews were conducted. Five were conducted in English, nine in Hindi and three in Marathi. During the interview, observations about the participants were made and written up after the session ended.

DATA ANALYSIS

The treatment and analysis of data followed the procedures elucidated by van Manen (1998). The purpose of phenomenological reflection is to grasp the essential meaning of something. The insight into the essence of a phenomenon involves a process of reflectively and appropriately clarifying and making explicit the structure of meaning of the lived experience. Meaning is multidimensional and multilayered, and can be best communicated through organised narrative or text. To carry out human science research is to be involved in the crafting of a text which describes the phenomenon in terms of themes (ibid.).

In defining themes, van Manen (1998) states that themes touch at the core of the notion we are trying to understand, helping us to make sense. Since they may not always completely unlock the enigmatic aspects of the experience, related sub-themes capturing details and nuances may be required to provide a comprehensive picture. The notion of theme implies making something of a lived experience by interpreting its meaning through a process of insightful invention, discovery or disclosure. Thematic analysis refers to the process of recovering the themes that are embodied or dramatised in the evolving meanings and imagery of the text.

Themes may be isolated through three approaches:

- A wholistic or sententious approach, where we attend to the text as a whole and capture its fundamental meaning.
- A selective or highlighting approach, where we repeatedly read/listen to the text and examine the meaning of statements which are particularly revealing.
- A detailed or line-by-line approach, where we study every sentence or sentence cluster to determine what it says about the experience (van Manen 1998).

In the present study, the attempt to isolate themes involved the first two approaches. Transcripts and field notes were read several times in order to gain a sense of the overall experience of the participant. Through the wholistic approach, the researcher tried to develop an idea of what it meant for a person to live the experience. Through this process, the researcher concluded that the lived experience for the three different groups of participants, namely, care receivers, seronegative caregivers and seropositive caregiving wives, was distinct. In other words, each group's experience had its own central meaning(s). The essence of care receivers' experiences were embodied in the key themes of losing autonomy and redefining family relationships. Seronegative caregivers' experiences are structured around the key theme of struggling to prolong the care receivers' life. The underlying meanings for caregiving wives were preserving family and learning whom to count on.

Following the identification of the essential theme, selective reading was undertaken, where significant statements, related to and illustrating the various dimensions of the essential theme, were identified and demarcated. These were read and re-read to formulate conceptual meanings and explore essential qualities of described experiences, and themes were identified in the process. As the themes emerged, the components of each participant's statements that were relevant for each meaning unit were highlighted. Redundancies in the units were eliminated and relevant statements were clustered.

Finally, for each group of participants, the core theme and their constituent themes were joined into a text that captured lived experience in its completeness. Chapters 4, 5 and 6 describe the lived experiences of care receivers, seronegative caregivers and seropositive caregivers, respectively.

Van Manen (1998) proposes formal or informal hermeneutic conversations with other researchers on key themes and themes in order to generate deeper insights. Themes are examined, articulated, reinterpreted, added, omitted and reformulated. The attempt is to derive a common orientation to the experience and to help the researcher see limits in his/her present vision and to transcend them. A collaborative rather than competitive stance is indispensable here. Realising the significance of this process for incorporating methodological rigour in the research, the researcher followed it in all the data analysis phases. Core themes, emerging conceptual categories and themes were discussed and critiqued with research colleagues, professional caregivers and experts in qualitative research. Based on the emerging discourse, reformulations were made till a consensual validation was achieved.

4
Losing Autonomy and Redefining Family Relationships

There were seven male care receivers who participated in the study. All of them were in the symptomatic stage of HIV infection, with four of them having been infected through the sexual mode. Of these, one was an intravenous drug user (IVDU). The age of the participants ranged from 26–36 years, with all except one having received some formal education, and all except one being employed/in business. Three of the care receivers belonged to upper-class families, two to lower-class families, and one each to lower-middle and middle-income groups. Two were receiving care in quasi-family contexts, four in traditional family contexts and one had the experience of both settings. In addition, five participants were in residential care at the time of the interview, though all of them had received/continued to receive familial care. Of these, four were in an institution for HIV-positive people and one was in a drug rehabilitation centre (see Table 4.1).

Care receiver narratives highlighted that the essential structure of their experience was captured in two themes: losing autonomy and redefining family relationships.

Losing Autonomy

Losing autonomy refers to participants' feeling that their lives are no longer in their hands following the seropositive diagnosis. Care receivers felt this way because of the anticipation of death, given the irreversibility of the diagnosis and because of the dependence

Table 4.1
Profile of care receivers

Participant	Gender	Age	Education	Occupation	Marital status/ No. of children	Present health status (symptom level)	Reported mode of infection	Caregiver/ family context	Co-residence with caregiver	Whether in residential care	HH income at the time of data collection (per month)
1	Male	34	SSC	Unemployed	Unmarried	Mild	Sexual	Initially family of origin, no origin, later friends / Traditional and later quasi-family	Yes for family, later for friends	No	10,500
2	Male	28	8th	Waiter/ bartender	Unmarried	Severe	Sexual	Mother / Traditional	Yes	Yes	36,000
3	Male	30	6th	Private driver	Separated	Severe	Suspected to be sexual	Brother / Traditional	No	Yes	2,800
4	Male	36	7th	Sells vegetables for owner	Unmarried	Moderate	Sexual	Mother / Traditional	Yes	Yes	20,600
5	Male	33	–	Temporary worker	Widowed/1	Severe	Not known	Employer / Quasi-family	No	Yes	1,200
6	Male	26	5th	Temporary worker	Unmarried	Moderate	Sexual	Friends / Quasi-family	Yes	No	1,000
7	Male	33	BA drop-out	Business	Separated/1	Mild	IVDU-sexual and/or parenteral	Mother Sister / Traditional	Yes	Yes	More than 12,000 but would not specify

on others, engendered by the progressive debilitation of the infection. Their feelings need to be looked at in the context of participants' developmental stage of adulthood, where independence is prized and where one perceives oneself as being on the threshold of fulfilling one's dreams and aspirations. The stigmatising nature of HIV created numerous limitations. The effects of indiscriminate disclosure on the part of testing centres and of the spread of the participants' serostatus resulted in changes in their social networks, while restrictions on the choice of treatment centres compromised participants' sense of control over their lives. Maintaining secrecy was a challenge that preoccupied care receivers and curtailed them in many ways.

The experience of losing autonomy began when care receivers heard about their seropositive diagnosis. For seropositive individuals, knowledge of their diagnosis was a turning point. Since all of them were already symptomatic at the time, it made a lot of difference to their perception of their health problem and their ways of coping with it. Prior to the knowledge of the diagnosis, illness episodes were considered to be inconsequential, passing phases and not much significance was attached to them. However, once the HIV status was known, it coloured participants' perception of their ill-health. Realising the gravity of the situation and its implications, care receivers experienced acute distress. Emotional strain emerged largely due to the stigmatising and terminal nature of the infection.

> I was so shocked to hear that I had this illness. The whole world seemed to collapse around me. Earlier, though I used to fall ill, it was different. I used to think that it would just pass off, but now ... I was terrified that people would reject me, I would suffer a lot, I would never get well ... I was not ready to die ... everything seemed so bleak, so hopeless. Earlier, there was always hope. (Nirav[1])

The prolonged and debilitating character of the infection contributed to their stress.

> I think about the progress of the disease—to be a patient in need of care, always sick, always in pain ... for so long ...

---

[1] All names are fictitious to maintain confidentiality.

then being unable to move, to do things for oneself .... And I am afraid—I have seen others in that condition and I do not want to be like that, suffering so much and making my family suffer along with me ... it is a horrible feeling .... (Jivan)

The terminal prognosis and its irreversibility represented grave blows to the care receivers. All of them nurtured aspirations and plans for themselves and had anticipated fulfilling these over the course of a normal life span. Hearing the fatal prognosis created a sense of doom and hopelessness. Participants realised that they might not be able to live out their hopes and plans, but would be at the mercy of the virus. According to them, hearing the diagnosis made them feel completely destroyed. They felt that they still had a lot of unfinished business in their lives, and hence the HIV virus cutting them short in their prime was seen as unfair. Moreover, there was a unanimous idea among all the care receivers that regardless of the treatment they underwent, the prognosis would not change, since there was no cure.

When I heard the diagnosis, it was as if time stopped for me ... I was so shocked and so stunned. I just cried and cried. Here, I was planning my future, I had so many dreams ... business, house, marriage, family ... and then I got this news. It was as if my life was no longer in my hands but someone else was calling the shots ... it is so unfair, I have hardly seen life, I have so much to do ... but it is all gone now because of this AIDS. (Nirav)

Except for one care receiver, none of the others, nor their caregivers/families could afford/were willing to undertake the expenses associated with anti-retroviral treatment to stall the progress of the infection. Care receivers acknowledged that they were in difficult circumstances, since on the one hand they wanted to stall the progress of the infection, but on the other hand, they could not avail of medications that could facilitate this process. A feeling of being trapped was reported.

I really have no alternatives ... living longer means taking those expensive medicines (anti-retrovirals), but where is the money for that? The doctors say I need 1000 rupees every day for it, so it is out of the question. (Manoj)

Yet, participants clung to the idea that a cure could be found and that if they were alive at that time, they would avail of it.

I still have hope that there will be a cure, some remedy for this horrible illness and then if I am still there (alive), I will be saved. It is a great hope that I have. (Jaideep)

Nonetheless, the anticipation of pain and suffering in the future, as the infection progressed, plagued most care receivers. They predicted a period of constant illness and severe symptoms that would restrict their mobility and possibly confine them to their beds. Being dependent on and burdensome to their caregivers were seen as logical fallouts, and anticipating them furthered participants' misgivings.

Adjusting to a position of dependence and of little or no autonomy over one's life during adulthood did not appear to be easy for them. Such experiences were perceived as out of synchrony with their development stage. Care receivers expressed dismay that at a time when they should have been in charge of their lives and providing for others, they were prolonging their childhood.

I do not like being ill and sitting idle, having everyone do things for me. I want to be independent and to do things for myself. At my age, I should be looking after others, doing things for my brother (who was looking after him) and his family. But instead, they have to look after me. They have to come with me to the doctor, get my medicines, give me my food, my sister-in-law has to wash my clothes ... instead of seeing to their family, they have to run after me. I feel ashamed of this. (Jaideep)

During the initial illness episodes which were of limited duration and alternated with 'well' periods, participants were able to accept their care receiving status more easily. However, once they knew the diagnosis and the chronic and prolonged nature of the infection and/or the severity increased, they did not take easily to their condition, resenting their recurrent needs for care and their dependence.

First when I was falling ill, it was OK ... meaning that Seth (his employer who looked after him) used to take me to the doctor, get my medicines, see my condition, but I would get well soon and be back on my feet, so I did not think much about it ... one or two, maximum four days being ill. But now it is different—the illness just goes on for months and then troubling Seth like that, I do not like it at all .... (Manoj)

In addition, discomfort for two care receivers arose because their caregivers were their elderly mothers, who themselves needed support due to age-related health problems. Care receivers felt deeply disturbed that at a time when they should be supporting their mothers, the latter were going through the strain of providing them with care. The role reversal resulted in feelings of awkwardness, guilt and shame.

I feel so bad that Ma (mother) has to do so much for me in her old age. She has so many health problems of her own— her eyes give her a lot of trouble so she has difficulty moving about. But instead of me doing for her, she has to look after me, come with me to the doctor, give me medicines, wash my clothes ... I feel so ashamed that a grown man like me is making his aged mother go through such physical strain. (Ajit)

One care receiver who had a history of drug abuse was troubled by his prolonged dependence and demands on his family.

My family has been helping me out for a very long time. They have stood by me throughout my drug habit. I have troubled them so much—robbed them, lied to them, cheated them, but still they care and they have spent so much on my treatment for so long. And now I have HIV—so it is an even greater burden for them. I feel very ashamed to keep troubling them. (Jivan)

Moreover, as care receivers became incapacitated, the inability to reciprocate the caregiver added to their feeling of discomfort.

All these feelings had consequences for the process of care receiving. They inhibited care receivers from accessing care and support. Care receivers were seen to postpone seeking support as far as possible.

> How much to go on troubling others? I keep asking myself that because this illness just goes on and on ... very often to feel better, I try to delay my demands. I wait for as long as I can before I ask for anything ... at least that way I don't feel so bad about myself. Of course, if it (my need) cannot be postponed or postponing it means damage to my health, then I ask for what I need. But if it can (be deferred), then I wait as much as possible. (Vivek)

Four care receivers had no control over the disclosure of their diagnosis. Healthcare professionals from certain public and private healthcare agencies where participants underwent testing violated testing guidelines and shared the infected person's serostatus with family members, without the HIV-positive person's knowledge and/or consent. The infected individual was made aware of his diagnosis from these people.

> I had severe diarrhoea which was not getting well. So I went to Hospital B (a public hospital in Mumbai), they admitted me. Without informing me, they did the AIDS test. And even when the result came, they did not inform me. They asked me to call my home people, and they told them. It is from my home people that I came to know I had AIDS. (Ajit)

The participant's choice, as to whether he would like to share the diagnosis or not, and thereby handle issues of confidentiality and stigma on his own, was thus pre-empted.

Though for all the four care receivers, the secrecy of their diagnosis was maintained by their family members, negative reactions on the part of some relatives in three instances made participants realise how dearly the loss of their confidentiality had cost them. The healthcare system, by sharing their seropositive diagnosis and allowing it to spread in the family, had exposed the positive individuals to stigmatising experiences that they would have taken care to guard themselves against, had they enjoyed autonomy and confidentiality over their diagnosis.

I wish that they (the personnel in Hospital B) had never said anything to my family—they mentioned the diagnosis to my brother and mother, (but) that is fine because they still accept me. But they told my sister-in-law also and she now behaves badly with me. She does not let me enter the house—I stay in the veranda, she gives me only one meal a day, I cannot watch TV (television). And she keeps tabs over how much is spent on me, giving only little money, so it is difficult for my mother to help me as much as she would like to or as much as I require, since she (mother) is dependent on her (sister-in-law). Left to myself, I would have thought twice about sharing the information, but now what to do? (Ajit)

Anger towards personnel in the errant agencies was obvious, but co-existed with resignation and a feeling that nothing could be done, not just because the damage had already taken place, but because it was believed that fighting doctors and nurses whom one was dependent on for treatment and who belonged to a powerful system, was futile.

See, we need the doctors and nurses—we have to turn to them only. So what can be done? There are such limited centres treating people like us that if we take up such matters we will be left with no options because these hospital people are all in one network together and they have lots of money and power. And in any case, now that it has happened, we should just move on. (Girish)

Having control over the spread of their diagnosis spelt great relief for three care receivers who enjoyed the confidentiality of their serostatus. Out of these, two participants had been tested in public-sector hospitals and one in an NGO. Personnel in these agencies had shared the diagnosis only with the infected individual, who could then decide whether to disclose it or not, and if so, with whom.

This AIDS is such that people keep away, they talk badly about you. So I was happy that the doctor told only me about my illness and not my friends who were with me. Then it was upto me to decide to tell them or no. Otherwise, I have heard that the doctors leak out the information and then the person with AIDS undergoes lots of problems—people stop talking, they throw you out of your job and so on. (Nirav)

All three care receivers stated that their immediate response was to guard the secrecy of their serostatus in order to protect themselves from discrimination. They were afraid of rejection, stigmatisation and isolation.

My first reaction was … I do not want to tell anybody. If people come to know, they will not let me live, they will look down on me. People will just gossip … treat me like an outcast. It is better to keep quiet about it. Why create problems for myself and for my family? (Jivan)

Yet, the emotional turmoil created by the knowledge and implications of a positive diagnosis, and the burden of secrecy which created feelings of isolation were so strong that all three were found to reveal the diagnosis to their caregivers in order to receive some psychological comfort and support.

Initially, my HIV diagnosis was known only to me. I did not want to tell my mother and sister. But keeping it to myself, it had become too much for me to bear on my own. I was getting depressed, suicidal …. So I thought that if I shared it with my mother and sister, it would help me. They are very close to me and I knew that they would be understanding and that I could trust them, so I did not mind telling them, they would still accept me and protect me. So I decided to tell them and when I did, they were, as I had predicted, supportive … they were very upset, of course, but they told me not to worry, they would make sure about the treatment and all … and so I felt less upset, less alone. (Jivan)

It was clear from the narratives that care receivers' decision to disclose their condition was not arbitrary. When they realised the intensity of their need, they objectively judged their caregiver/ social support system and the advantages and disadvantages of disclosing their seropositive status. They realised that their caregivers' personality was responsible for the great trust that they had in them, and both these factors led them to believe that the chances of rejection and compromise were few. On the contrary, they would gain support which would help them cope. This realisation clinched their decision. Indeed, none of their confidants let them down and sharing the information was found to bring great solace and connectedness for all care receivers. Confidants themselves took great pains to maintain secrecy.

Care receivers lacked the privilege of choosing the place where they could receive treatment, on account of the discriminatory practices of many healthcare personnel and many organisations in the public and private health sectors. Prior to diagnosis, the HIV-infected individuals were free to pursue whatever treatment they wished, from any part of the healthcare system they chose. However, once the HIV diagnosis was made, most treatment centres in both the public and private health sectors refused to treat them and redirected them to specific public-sector hospitals (viz., Hospitals A, B, C and D) and NGO centres (viz., NGOs A, B and C).

I was diagnosed in a private nursing home near my place. Since I had been falling ill for sometime before the test, I had been going to a private doctor near my home. Then when I was very ill and weak, my brother and sister-in-law admitted me to a private nursing home near our place. But when I was found to have AIDS, the nursing home people told me to go to Hospital A for treatment—they said that there was nothing further they could do, they did not handle such cases and so I should go to Hospital A. The nurses over there told my brother that it was better to go directly to Hospital A rather than anywhere else since other places would also refuse to treat such a disease. (Jaideep)

This discriminatory response limited the care and support options of the positive people. As a result, they had fewer agencies to choose from and some of them, along with their caregivers, were forced to travel long distances, at high indirect costs and physical strain, even during advanced stages of the infection, to access treatment.

After the diagnosis, we started going to Hospital A only for treatment. Though it is located at the end of the city and is so far from our place, my brother said that we should go there only, after what we had been told by the staff of the nursing home (where testing had taken place). So we went over there, but it is so far that when I am weak, I cannot go on my own, someone, either my brother or sister-in-law, have to come with me, which means that their schedule gets interrupted. But my brother would worry that with my physical condition and the strain of travelling, it was not advisable for me to go alone. And then, you know how expensive travelling in Mumbai is—that too, if there are two of us. (Jaideep)

HIV-seropositive participants, looking to the healthcare system for support, reported feelings of being wronged. However, as mentioned earlier, behaviourally they remained resigned, putting down these experiences as their fate. Their passivity arose not only because they were unaware of avenues of redressal, but also because they knew that they were dependent on doctors and nurses for healthcare and because they perceived the system as too powerful and invincible for them to fight successfully.

In any case, the clinical intervention offered by select public health sector centres practising allopathy (Hospitals A, B and C) was seen as unreliable. Though medical treatment was free of cost, participants were unhappy with staff behaviour and attitudes, and with the infrastructure and services. Personnel were perceived as too busy, too curt and/or too indifferent. Diagnostic facilities were often in a broken-down condition, while medicines were not always in stock in the dispensary. As a result, they had to wait for the services, make their own arrangements or do without them.

First of all, they say that we can go to only some hospitals and then there too you cannot get quality treatment—these government hospitals are supposed to be free but most of the time, you cannot get medicines or tests cannot be done because the machine is out of order—so it causes problems with the treatment because if you cannot afford to get things done outside (in private health centres), then you have to just manage without the service. So how can you maintain your health? Most of the time, the doctors will not even take five minutes to explain the dosage, so you are never sure of how you are taking the medicines. (Ajit)

Similar hardships were reported in relation to centres providing homoeopathic services for HIV/AIDS as well (Hospitals B and D). Two of the participants availed of homoeopathic services since these were recommended by their allopathic doctors as beneficial in stalling the progress of the infection. However, these facilities were also located in specific public hospitals, entailing a great deal of travel. Consultation was provided free of cost, as were medicines if they were available in the dispensary. Indirect costs, particularly travel time and expense, were high, while purchasing medicines privately was economically unfeasible. Thus, even though the contribution of alternative systems of medicine to health status was reported to be beneficial, impediments to compliance existed.

> Homoeopathic medicine was effective—I took it for a while and my doctor found that it halted progress of the illness. But often the medicines were unavailable in the hospital and had to be bought privately. I could not afford this over an extended period of time because the treatment is a long-drawn one, so I stopped it. (Ajit)

Though public-sector health centres did provide some services to the care receivers, the problems associated with them exacerbated participants' sense of helplessness. The difficulties in obtaining and continuing treatment raised doubts in their minds as to whether they could stall the progress of the infection and maintain their health.

Intervention from the voluntary sector was evaluated favourably. The services provided here, which went beyond medical treatment to include emotional support, material assistance and networking with other agencies, were given free of cost by sensitive personnel and were consistently available. Care receivers knew that they could rely on these organisations and that they were steadily available throughout their struggle. The attitude of the personnel not only comforted them but also made them feel valued and respected. Yet, the support of the voluntary sector posed a dilemma for the care receiving participants. While they appreciated it as a source of support and as a pleasant and reassuring change from the rejection and discrimination of the public and private sectors, they perceived themselves as dependent on the voluntary sector.

Two care receivers were receiving emotional, medical and network support from NGO A on an out-patient department (OPD) basis, while five participants were in residential care. Also, four participants were living in a residential facility for HIV/AIDS (NGO C) while one was undergoing an in-house drug rehabilitation programme (NGO B). Residential care for HIV/AIDS was opted for under a variety of circumstances such as: quasi-familial contexts, where caregivers had ceased to provide care (one); care receiver's disappointment at the limited care provided at home (one); and as a stop-gap arrangement until the opportunistic infection of tuberculosis (TB) subsided in the seropositive person (two).

While care receivers gained information about NGO C through the operation of network support either from formal (two) or informal (two) sources, the decision to transfer care from the family to the institution was made by the seropositive person only in the cases of the quasi-family context and limited care. In the cases of seropositive individuals suffering from TB, the decision was made jointly by the family caregiver and the care receiver.

Clinical treatment, medicines and material support such as food and shelter were provided free of cost at NGO C by trained staff. Participants spoke appreciatively about the quality of care that they received. Further, the therapeutic value of the agency's geographical location and physical surroundings was described. The fresh air, greenery, silence and open environment away from the city soothed them. Though they were not ordinarily allowed to go out of the premises, the compound was large enough for them to walk around in, if their physical condition permitted. The group nature of the facility was also therapeutic, though it was not designed with that intention. Positive people living here were able to cope better and overcome some of their distress when they saw that others too were suffering like they were and that they were not alone. Learning from the experiences of others, soliciting their suggestions, gaining and giving support, in particular emotional support, worked in a positive way.

I feel this place (NGO C) is good. One gets nutritious food, on time. Medicines are also given on time. The staying facilities are comfortable—location is also good, clean, fresh air, trees, no noise. Everything is free. Sisters (nuns in charge) are very good—they serve us very well. Anything one wants,

any problem you tell them, they will see to it, give medicines and always ask about one's health. If one is upset,
they give a lot of comfort. They come—the older sister comes
twice a day and the young sister comes four times a day. If
anyone comes to know that this person has HIV, they will
never come near but the sisters come near, they touch us.
Seeing other patients has also been helpful—we share our
experiences and encourage each other, we do things for each
other. (Jaideep)

While their experiences at NGO C evoked satisfaction which
co-existed with a sense of dependence, comparisons with family
care were inevitable. Where family care was whole-hearted and
unconditional, it was sorely missed.

This place (NGO C) is good, no doubt. But I do not want to
be here. I want to be at home—there is no place like home
and family, and my family cares so much and so nicely for
me. I miss them, but what to do—there are small children
in the house and they could get my TB so we cannot take
the risk. (Jaideep)

However, if the response from the family was mixed, as reported by two care receivers, in that some members limited the
care that they provided while others did their best to support the
HIV-positive family member, participants were divided in their
opinions. The first preferred institutional care since there was
consistency and punctuality in the provision of care.

At home, my sister-in-law limits the care I get even though
my mother would like to give me a lot—of course within her
constraints, my mother does her best. But compared to my
situation at home where I have to stay in the balcony and
get just one meal from home, and have to arrange for the
other meal myself, this place (NGO C) is very good because
I can rest comfortably, get all my meals without any
problem—people are very supportive and warm. Generally,
things can be taken for granted here while at home, one can
never be sure—my sister-in-law's wishes play an important
role. (Ajit)

The other care receiver preferred being cared for at home, despite the hostility from some quarters.

> My sister-in-law is cold towards me—she is upset with me for getting this illness and causing problems for the family. So she just gives me the basic things. My mother depends on her (sister-in-law) for money and she gives her very little. So it is actually a difficult situation at home. But still, I would prefer to be looked after at home by my mother, because then I would get personalised care and attention. Mummy would see to every detail and every need and do things exactly as I like them because she knows me so well and cares for me. (Girish)

All these participants realised, at the same time, that residential care was a boon to their caregivers since the latter were relieved, to a large extent at least for the time being, of the execution of caregiving tasks, giving them some respite, while simultaneously being reassured that their loved one was well looked after.

> Now I am here (NGO C) so it is good for my mother. She can visit my sister and stay with her—otherwise, she has to be at home to see to me because my sister-in-law does not bother much. And since my mother comes with me to the doctor, gives me my medicines, washes my clothes ... like that ... she is a bit tied up. Now she is free and it is a break from the strenuous work too ... being looked after here means my mother need not worry about me. (Ajit)

In quasi-family contexts (one), where care had ceased after it became too demanding, residential care was seen as a saving grace for those who had no family to look after them.

> When I became severely ill, then after a point my Seth (employer who was looking after him) said, 'I cannot look after you anymore ... if I look after you, I will have no time to look after the business.' Now I have no family, no one, so where could I go? Who would help me? Places like this (NGO C) are the best for me. (Manoj)

Overall, the knowledge of the seropositive diagnosis altered the care receivers' lives irrevocably. Participants stated that they could no longer live their lives freely and on their own terms. They had to take care not to transmit the infection, not to exert themselves, and had to be always careful about their lifestyle and behaviour. Maintaining secrecy and limiting the spread of the infection was an important consideration too. The anticipation of death and a shortened lifespan caused deep regret. Relinquishing their long cherished aspirations precipitated distress. In this new reality, HIV was reported as being almost always at the back of their minds.

REDEFINING FAMILY RELATIONSHIPS

Notwithstanding their discomfort with the care receiving role, all care receivers were receiving care within a family/quasi-family context, and their evaluations of the care and support that they received influenced the way they perceived their caregivers and their families. These perceptions affected care receivers' interactions with, and manner of relating to, their caregivers and family members. To state things simply, where care receivers were happy with the care they were receiving, existing good relations were strengthened, while tenuous relations improved. Dissatisfaction with the care provided led to either worsening of already poor relations, or severing ties with the family.

Care receiver narratives brought out the complex dynamics surrounding the changes. For two care receivers whose caregiving system comprised a dyad of their mothers and sisters-in-law, a differential response to each member of the dyad was observed, contingent on the care provided by each caregiver. Within the dyad, an unequal relationship prevailed. Elderly mothers provided care through the actual execution of caregiving tasks, though they depended on their daughters-in-law (the care receiver's sister-in-law) for the resources to do so. The daughters-in-law, because of their economic power, influenced the decisions about care, and since they harboured negative feelings towards the seropositive individuals for their lifestyles due to which they contracted HIV and brought problems for the family, they decided to limit the care provided. The mothers who wished to provide the best possible care, despite acknowledging the son's past lifestyle, found themselves constrained due to their lack of resources.

> My sister-in-law is very upset with me for having got this disease. She feels that I have caused a lot of problems for the family, because first of all, if others get to know, it will be a big problem. Moreover, she and my brother run the house with their money so they have to undertake the expenses for my treatment and that also makes her very upset. She goes on grumbling about this but then she has to look after me, no choice about it, so she does the minimum. She gives my mother very little money, tries to make sure that expenditure for me is minimised, so my mother gets very upset but then what to do? My mother is dependent on them—my mother feels very bad, because on account of these people and the limited money that they give her, she cannot do as much as she would like for me. (Girish)

Care receivers responded differently to both the caregiving women. Observing the efforts of the mothers to provide optimal care despite their age, and the attitude of and constraints presented by the sisters-in-law, resulted in feelings of appreciation and admiration from the sons. Moreover, sons realised that mothers were able to transcend their negative feelings about the former's earlier lifestyle and tenuous filial relationships and provide care. They acknowledged the difficult circumstances under which their mothers were providing care and admired their ability to manage a multiplicity of challenges. They were also touched by their mother's generosity of spirit and selfless attitude, and thus related to them with affection and gratitude.

> Earlier, my relationship with my mother was full of conflicts—I used to fight with her. I would tell her, 'What have you done for us?' And she would get upset with me because I used to drink, gamble, disappear for days on end ... so there were a lot of problems between us. But in spite of that, she is looking after me. She knows that because of my earlier behaviour this disease has come, but she has never scolded me or reprimanded me ... I know she feels upset

about it but still she does her best to help me. My sister-in-law's behaviour has made things so tough for her like she has to look after me with little money so she cannot do whatever she wants to do ... she has to see about my food, washing my clothes, come with me to the doctor, like that. That too, she is old, with so many problems of her own, but she never lets that interfere with looking after me. It is a very tough situation for her and I admire the way she manages—even in her position putting me first. Our whole relationship has changed because of this—we have become very close. We now speak to each other a lot more, we get along well, share our concerns, I do things for her—take her for her check-ups, get things she wants to eat, we spend time together. (Ajit)

Care receivers resented the attitude of their sisters-in-law and the limited care that they provided. They felt that the latter should put in greater efforts to help them, particularly when they had the means to do so. However, at the same time, care receivers acknowledged that it was difficult to blame their sisters-in-law for their negative feelings, since their lifestyles had been very difficult and problematic for their families and had finally resulted in grave consequences given the features of the HIV infection and the costs it entailed. Nonetheless, care receivers' empathy with their sisters-in-law and their acknowledgement that, notwithstanding their negative feelings, they did not reject them altogether, could not obliterate their sense of bitterness over the limited care being provided. Care receivers were therefore seen to minimise their interactions with the sisters-in-law.

Well, it is true that my behaviour was not good—going out, drinking, gambling ... but now I am at death's door and when she (sister-in-law) can afford to help me out with better care, she will not. I keep asking myself why she cannot forgive me and help me out more. Of course, I guess I should be happy that she is helping me out at all but I feel very bad, very angry about her attitude—after all, just because she is upset, I have to suffer more. Can't she try and understand my situation? I even find it difficult to relate to her because of all this. (Girish)

Another care receiver whose entire blood family blamed him for contracting HIV and causing problems for them, rejected the limited care they were providing. He turned to his friends instead. The generous support he received from his friends made the bonds between them stronger.

> When I was ill, they (my family) would look after me. But all the time, they would keep taunting me, saying, 'Half the time you are jobless, you are going out to joints, then you keep falling sick.' So I decided that I did not want to hear all this anymore, and I refused to take anything from them. I ask my friends to help me when I am ill and they willingly come forward. I do not accept anything from them (family). (Vivek)

Two other seropositive individuals in quasi-family situations were also found to display a lot of appreciation for the care they received. Being provided care in the absence of a blood/marital bond made care receivers very grateful for what they received. They were happy that someone was looking after them, because basically they had no blood/marital family who was obliged to undertake the responsibility. Therefore, even though caregivers in these cases ceased providing care after a point of time (when caregiving became too demanding), care receivers remained positive in their evaluations and displayed no bitterness. From their narratives, it was obvious that they shared a relationship of attachment with their caregivers.

> He (my employer) did a lot for me, though he didn't have to. He paid for my treatment, took to me doctors, admitted me to hospital, visited me in hospital, provided me with food and living space. He undertook all this without telling me the costs or asking for anything in return. I am indebted to him. And I don't hold it against him that he stopped—after all, he was not obliged to care for me. And when it got too much, he felt that it was interfering with his work and his family. Yet he did so much because he had regard for me as I was one of his best and most hardworking and reliable workers. But how much can he do? One's own family is a different issue, but I have no one, so I cannot expect beyond a point. So even what he did was too much for me, I feel.

Despite his position and responsibility, he did for me—it was a great thing for me. And even now, if I visit him, he gives me money, food. (Manoj)

Caregiver and care receiver bonding enhanced care receivers' experiences of emotional support. For the care receivers, they felt that someone was there for them at a time of deep distress, and the perception of connectedness helped them to feel less alone.

In such situations, care receivers were seen to demonstrate concern towards their caregivers. Observing the strain that the performance of the caregiving role engendered and how it disrupted the caregivers' life, care receivers expressed feelings of sadness, shame and guilt at burdening the caregivers.

My being ill has been a real problem for my brother and sister-in-law. And I feel really guilty about it. After all, they have their own responsibilities and their own family—and that should be their priority, not me. Brother works long hours and his earnings are just enough for them—they want to buy a house, but instead, they had to use their savings for my treatment. The children are small—but to see to me, sister-in-law had to leave them with the neighbours or call her brother and sister to be with them. Then she has to manage all the housework. So it is quite hard for them. But they never once complain or make me feel unwanted or a burden ... I feel so ashamed that instead of standing on my own feet, I am putting them through this. (Jaideep)

Acknowledging their role in the process and empathising with their caregivers, care receivers attempted to cope with the situation by displaying sensitivity to the caregivers. Care receivers would minimise/postpone the demands they made on caregivers to the extent possible, and would demonstrate affection and emotional support towards them.

I always felt bad that my friends were inconvenienced because of me and having to look after me so I would try to manage as much as I could on my own and take their help only when it was unavoidable. (Nirav)

Where caregivers lacked economic resources, care receivers were aware of the financial drain (both direct and indirect) posed by their illness and of the consequent pressure on the caregiver and caregiving family to deal with the situation and to provide care in spite of it. Responding to the predicament of their caregivers, care receivers would forego certain things and adjust to their circumstances, as much as was possible.

> My brother is not rich and I know that in order to care for me, he has had to spend a lot—even his savings which he had accumulated to buy a house ... so he and his wife are depriving themselves and their family for me. So as far as possible, I always try to make do with what I have instead of asking them and making them spend more—I ask only when there is no other way out. (Jaideep)

Reciprocity was also uppermost in care receivers' minds, and all of them described how important it was to be able to repay their caregivers. Though demonstrating emotional support and concern formed an integral part of their relationship with their caregivers during the course of the illness trajectory, care receivers placed a greater value on reciprocating through tangible ways. This was seen as a more significant and more appropriate form of reciprocity, which would better demonstrate their appreciation for the care received and indicate that they understood the costs of care for the caregiver. Moreover, it was also seen as an avenue to assuage their discomfort and shame at being dependent. Thus, all care receivers had well thought out plans about how they could repay their caregivers in tangible terms when their current opportunistic infection/symptoms abated.

> When I get well, I will go back and work for Seth (the employer who had looked after him) and I will make sure that his business prospers—I will work tirelessly for him. He has done so much for me and this is the only way in which I can show him how much I appreciate his support. If I cannot do this, then I will always feel guilty and ashamed that I took so much and gave back nothing. (Manoj)

5

STRUGGLING TO PROLONG LIFE

The study included three female and two male seronegative caregivers whose ages ranged from 33–60 years. Of these, three caregivers were married with young/adolescent children, while one was widowed. The male caregivers held earner positions and one of them, a medical practitioner, was caring for two HIV-positive family members, unlike the other four caregivers, who provided care for one care receiver each. Further, one of the participants had lost her HIV-positive caregiver by the time of data collection, whereas for the other four caregivers, their care receivers were in various stages of symptomatic infection, except for one, who was asymptomatic. Two caregivers belonged to the upper-income group, while one caregiver each belonged to the middle, lower-middle and lower-income groups. The quasi-family context operated in one instance (see Table 5.1).

The essential core of caregivers' experiences centred around their struggle to prolong the life of their loved one. This relates to caregivers' endeavour to provide optimal care and extend the life of their HIV-infected family member(s) as much as possible, in spite of odds such as the stigmatising nature of the HIV infection, which restricts seeking support, the limited assistance from the healthcare system, paucity of economic resources, caregiver health status, and so on.

The perception of the caregiving role as being an attempt to prolong life began on hearing the terminal prognosis. Though all the care receivers except one were symptomatic prior to the knowledge of the diagnosis and hence caregiving was already underway, it was the prognosis of death that made caregivers redefine their caregiving role.

Table 5.1
Profile of seronegative caregivers

Participant	Gender	Age	Education	Occupation	Marital status/No. of children	Care receiver/ Family context	Co-residence with care receiver	Whether care receiver is/was in residential care	Suspected source of care receiver's infection	Care receiver's symptom level	HH income at the time of data collection (per month)
1	Female	60	–	Housewife	Widowed/5	Son Traditional	Yes	Yes	Sexual	Severe	36,000
2	Female	40	SSC	Housewife	Married/2	Son Traditional	Yes	No	Parenteral (Care receiver was thalassemic)	Moderate	6,000
3	Female	55	–	Brothel owner	Not known/2	Woman considered to be a daughter Quasi-family	Yes	No	Sexual	Deceased	500 to 1,000
4	Male	33	7th	Private driver	Married/2	Brother Traditional	Initially no, later yes	Yes	Sexual	Severe	2,800
5	Male	36	Medical graduate	General practitioner	Married/1	Brother and father Traditional	Yes	No	Brother– not known Father– parenteral	Brother– asympto- matic Father– mild	20,000

He (son) had been falling ill for a long while ... off and on, he would fall ill, get well. I did not think much of it at that time ... passed it off as part of the normal course of things. But when I heard of this deadly AIDS, then I realised how serious the situation was, that he would die. For me at that time, my role was not just about looking after him, it was about saving his life, about helping him live. (Anita, caregiving mother)

Caregivers were deeply distressed by the prospect of losing their family member, a response heightened in most cases by the developmental stage of the care receiver. The perception here was that the care receiver was too young to die.

When I heard that he (brother) had this illness, I was devastated. I did not eat for 2–3 days. I was so upset that we were going to lose him that I could not think properly. After all, he is my younger brother and I love him very much—losing him was unthinkable. And that too, he is so young, his life is just beginning—and before that, it has been nipped in the bud .... (Rohit, caregiving brother)

For parental caregivers, the pain of outliving their offspring was palpable.

In the normal course of life, parents pass away before their children. And this was exactly opposite. I could not even imagine my youngest son going before me—it was against Nature, against my dreams, against everything. I was so disturbed that I could not think straight for a few days after getting his diagnosis. (Anita, caregiving mother)

Caregivers began to regard their care receivers with an air of protectiveness, and caregiving became an attempt to fight the terminal prognosis and postpone death as much as possible. The advice of healthcare personnel that an infected individual who maintains his/her health can live for 10–20 years, reinforced caregivers' resolve.

The doctors told us that there was no cure for her (adopted daughter's) illness but if we looked after her health, she could live for 10–20 years. So this became our objective—to help her maintain her health and live as long as possible. That way, even if she eventually died of AIDS, we would have extended her life as much as we could. So we began to do whatever we could to help her. (Savitri, caregiving adopted mother)

As a result, caregivers began to work tirelessly towards prolonging the life of their loved one.

To help him (son) live means that nothing is enough—my husband and I leave no stone unturned. We keep doing our best for him, regardless of what it means for us. No matter how tired I am, if I feel that there is something to be done which can help him, I do it. (Sukanya, caregiving mother)

Indeed, this orientation helped an elderly caregiving mother, who in the past had been unhappy with her son's lifestyle and who attributed the contracting of HIV to his earlier behaviour, to overcome her anger and reproach, and to provide care wholeheartedly.

That he (son) was going to die and that I had to save his life is what made me forget about the past—I knew about his earlier ways of drinking, gambling, what not, and I used to always be angry with him about it because it is not good, it causes a lot of problems as it actually had with this AIDS. But then later, extending his life was a priority. So focusing on that made the past seem irrelevant. Seeing him as someone whom we could lose made me forget the earlier problems, made me single-mindedly focus on the task of helping him live. (Anita, caregiving mother)

Through their task-oriented approach, caregivers provided hands-on care in instances of severe illness and incapacitation, medical support through accompanying the person to treatment centres, supervising and administering medication and monitoring health status, healthy diet and lifestyle, as well as emotional support. Their goal was to help care receivers regain their asymptomatic state and lead a long life.

Prolonging the life of their loved one(s) was a driving force for the caregivers, but enmeshed in the process were numerous impediments that made the caregiving trajectory a struggle. Primary among these were the stigmatising nature of the HIV infection and the need to maintain secrecy. Though violations of confidentiality guidelines on the part of personnel in public and private healthcare centres had resulted in three caregivers and their families becoming aware of the seropositive diagnosis directly, they had to make sure that the diagnosis did not spread outside the household. They therefore had to rely on those within the household for support, influencing the organisation of care.

> My daughter-in-law does not really allow me to give him (son) the care that I would like to—she controls the expenditure and since I have no money of my own and have to take from her, I have no choice as such. But what to do? This illness is such that one cannot tell others about it—they will stay away, they will think badly about us, they will talk about us. So I cannot ask others for help also. I just have to manage with the house people. (Anita, caregiving mother)

One caregiver, looking after his seropositive brother, shared the responsibility equally with his wife, resulting in a partnership.

> My wife helps me a lot in caring for him (brother). In fact, we share it. Both of us take turns in going with him to the doctor, supervising his medicines ... she sees about his nutrition, I plan his treatment. So it is properly distributed between us. (Rohit, caregiving brother)

The caregiving adopted mother and two members of her household distributed caregiving tasks amongst themselves in a multiple caregiver arrangement.

> These two women and I used to look after her (adopted daughter). We would share the various tasks—feeding her, bathing her, taking her to the toilet, going with her to the hospital or to NGO D, giving her medicines. And plus, we would jointly see to the house, the cooking, to her child. (Savitri, caregiving adopted mother)

An elderly caregiving mother found herself in an unequal relationship with her daughter-in-law. Although the mother executed
caregiving tasks, she was financially dependent on her elder son
(who was seronegative) and his wife. The daughter-in-law, who
managed household finances, made the decisions about
caregiving and since she was angry with the care receiver for his
lifestyle which had resulted in his HIV-positive status, which in
turn caused problems for the family, she provided the minimum
financial support required for his care. Not only did the caregiving
mother find her efforts to do her best to extend her son's life
constrained as a result of her daughter-in-law's attitude, but also
the need to maintain the confidentiality of the diagnosis put limits on the mother's efforts to seek support from other sources. In
the process, providing the care that she wished to, proved to be
very difficult since she could not access appropriate and sufficient
resources.

> I want to do so much for him (son) but I have to depend on
> _____ (other son and his wife) for money. And she (other
> son's wife) is so angry with him for creating problems for us
> that she does not want to spend on him, just give him the
> minimum, so she restricts the cash that she gives me. So
> even though we can afford to give him better care, she refuses
> to do so. That leaves me with hardly any chance to do what
> I want ... it is so upsetting ... I try and save from the money
> she gives me to run the house but that is hardly anything.
> And with this illness, I cannot freely ask for help from others
> also, so it is very dissatisfying. (Anita, caregiving mother)

For two caregivers, whose care receiving family members did
not experience any unethical practices during the testing process,
sharing the diagnosis with a few family members was not seen as
a threat because of the nature of the relationship shared and the
extent of the trust enjoyed between the parties. As a result, both
caregivers (one, a primary caregiver, and the other, in a caregiving
partnership with her husband) received support for their roles.
However, there was a need to maintain secrecy beyond this group.

> When we (husband and I) got to know that he (son) was
> positive, that time my elder brother-in-law's children were

living with us. They were quite grown up and we were quite close to them and their parents, we knew their nature—so we told them. We were so upset that it was a relief to share it. And we knew that there was no problem in doing so—they would always stand by us. Moreover, they knew that he had this thalassemia and that is how he got HIV—it was not his fault or anything like that. They were living with us, so they knew his habits and all. Others may not understand—they will not bother about the thalassemia but only consider the AIDS and think badly of us or say that he did something and got it. But these people are not like that—they were very helpful. They would always comfort us, help us to look after him or help us with the housework if we were busy looking after him. Now they no longer live here but they are always very solicitous—they send us money or gifts, keep in touch by phone, inquire how things are. And when they come to Mumbai, they stay with us and help us out. (Sukanya, caregiving mother)

Maintaining secrecy made role performance difficult. Caregivers had to make up stories to cover up for their behaviour and for the predicament of their care receiver. They had to lie about the diagnosis and the line of treatment, while developing plausible stories about the chronic, progressively deteriorating illness.

Well, the neighbours do ask what is happening—why he (brother) is always ill, not getting better and so on. I guess it is natural that people inquire and wonder what is happening. But we just tell them that it is TB and that it was not detected in time and like that, we manage. (Rohit, caregiving brother)

There were also implications for need fulfilment and support seeking. While most of them could satisfy their needs within the social network which was aware of the diagnosis, there were instances where they had to seek support beyond this group. Soliciting support under circumstances of secrecy of the HIV diagnosis involved a series of carefully deliberated decisions, stemming from the fear generated by the stigmatising nature of the HIV infection. Caregivers meticulously weighed the pros and cons of whether they should seek out help. First, they evaluated their need to see if it demanded immediate attention or could be postponed. In other words, they were willing to put off attending to their needs until they became absolutely unavoidable. Once this was resolved, then based on what they actually required, they considered possible sources of support. Of these, they shortlisted those who were in the best position to help them out and from whom they were comfortable receiving support. The next thing to decide upon was whether support seeking should involve disclosure of the seropositive diagnosis or not. Depending on the need and/or whom they were accessing support from, caregivers decided what exactly they should say and whether they should disclose their care receiver's seropositive status during the process of soliciting assistance. More than anything else, the need they were seeking to satisfy dictated the necessity for disclosure. Some needs necessitated the disclosure of the care receiver's HIV status and caregivers had no choice but to comply.

> We (my wife and I) were looking for a place where we could keep him (brother) till his TB subsided. We felt that though HIV does not spread, TB does and since our children are small and the house is tiny, if he lives with us, they may get it. But we knew of no such place, so we decided to contact Father ____ (a priest known to the family) and Sister ____ (a nun known to the family), as they were the only ones who could help us. And since we were looking for something specific, we had to tell them that he had HIV. Even to tell them we felt bad. But what to do? That way they are such great people, we knew that they would never turn against us and they did not. Of course not. That is why we did not mind approaching them, but still we felt bad. (Rohit, caregiving brother)

Where the need was not so specific and could be fulfilled by a number of people, a different process operated. If families could trust the person from whom they were seeking support with the secrecy of the diagnosis and be sure that he/she would help them without being judgemental, soliciting support was accompanied by disclosure, even if it was not needed or asked for and could have been avoided. If, on the other hand, they were not sure how the person would react, they would cover up their need for support with a plausible excuse, refusing to take the risk of being truthful. A process of discernment was thus apparent.

See, I will approach those who I will benefit from. And I will ask them for help. Now whether I tell them the diagnosis or not, depends. My family will help in looking after, but I will not tell them the diagnosis because they will collapse, they may refuse to care. But I'll tell them such that they will take precautions. With my professional friends, I can rely on them for medical and emotional support, and they will keep it confidential. So I can tell them the diagnosis. With my religious friends, I go for emotional support and I'll tell them it is a deadly illness. That would suffice. (Arvind, caregiving brother and son)

Reluctance to solicit support and fear of disclosing the care receiving family member's HIV-seropositivity were very clearly seen even in instances where the care receiver was said to be 'innocently' infected and was not seen as personally responsible for contracting the HIV infection. A caregiver looking after a thalassemic seropositive adolescent who had been parenterally infected through blood transfusions, was hesitant to access support from the social network and did not see disclosure as an option.

We (husband and I) have not told anyone, except his (husband's) elder brother and his family, about his (son's) HIV infection. Our other relatives like my parents and brothers and sisters, and his sisters—we did not tell them. People may or may not understand, you never know. And if we tell and by chance it slips from their mouths to others, then our entire community will come to know, and not everyone will be good and understanding. Even though he has been infected due to a blood transfusion, and everyone knows he is a thalassemic, once they are told he has this AIDS, one never knows how people's minds will work—they may just insist that he has done something wrong and then reject us. So instead of having that tension, it is better to keep it to ourselves and manage on our own. Of course, I feel it—the loneliness and pain are so acute, particularly now that my brother-in-law and his family have moved out of the country. I sometimes feel that it would be a relief to share with my people. But the risk always remains, so we feel it is better to stay silent. What I tell you so easily and (in the

process), experience so much relief, I cannot tell anyone.
(Sukanya, caregiving mother)

The general consensus was that the stigmatising nature of the HIV infection impeded effective caregiving when caregivers needed to look for assistance beyond the limited social circle who were aware of the diagnosis.

Though all the caregivers sought to do their best for their HIV-infected family member(s), they were aware that their economic resources posed/could pose a constraint and this was found to disturb them. The elderly caregiving mother referred to earlier was from an upper-income group family, but her economic dependence limited the resources she had at her disposal since she had to rely on her daughter-in-law for money. The daughter-in-law, blaming the care receiver for causing problems for the family, did not wish to spend money on his treatment, even though she had the resources to do so. She therefore provided the minimum support required for his care. To supplement this, the mother would try and save from her household allowance or forego some of her own needs, but refrained from accessing support from others because of the stigmatising nature of the HIV infection and the need to maintain confidentiality. Economic resources were insufficient for the mother to provide the kind of care that she wished to. Though she ensured that she did her best within the constraints of her circumstances, from her story it was clear that the inadequate support and lack of co-operation from her family made her feel lonely in her struggle against the virus, besides creating a sense of indignation that though resources were available, they were being denied out of anger over past behaviour. It was beyond her comprehension as to why her daughter-in-law could not soften her stand and forgive the infected family member, when his diagnosis itself was sufficient punishment for him. In her opinion, her daughter-in-law should at least realise that the son's last days should be made as pleasant as possible. Since that had not happened and the mother had to provide care without the appropriate means to do so, she was greatly distressed.

I really want to help my son, I want him to live but it seems so difficult for me ... my daughter-in-law is adamant about the spending and I have no resources of my own. I cannot turn to anyone either, so it is a very lonely experience, very sad ... I wish she would understand that this is our last chance to help him out but she won't relent. I mean, when his life is hanging like this, how can she go on being angry about his past? I just cannot imagine .... What to do? I try my best—stinge on the house expenses, let go of things that I can do without and try to manage the best possible. (Anita, caregiving mother)

Three caregivers with modest means reported using whatever resources they had to help out their seropositive loved one, even though this often meant sacrificing the needs of other family members. For instance, one caregiver from a lower-middle-income group household considered his HIV-positive brother's life to be very precious and hence decided to spend the money he had struggled to save to purchase a house for his brother's care.

I want to do a lot for him (brother)—I want him to live. But I do not have that much of money. As a driver, I do not earn that much. So I had to adjust somewhere and the money I saved for years to buy a house—I used it up for his treatment, but never mind, his life has to be protected so if I have some means, I will use it. (Rohit, caregiving brother)

Another caregiver from the lower-income group stated that while the care receiving family member was given top priority in intra-household resource distribution, regardless of the needs of other family members, getting support from NGO D supplemented limited family resources so that better care could be provided. Since this support, which included assistance with medical treatment, nutrition and aid for the education of the care receiver's child, took care of some of the care receiving woman's needs, household resources could be reallocated to cover her other needs, improving the quality and quantity of care provided.

Money is a problem for us—we do not have so much. But because we wanted to do our best for her (adopted daughter) so that she could live, we used whatever we had for her. She always came first. Our needs did not matter—we would ignore them. Since we wanted to do so much but had so little, the help from NGO D was a blessing for us. Because we were getting help from there for her food, medicines, her son's food and education, we could use our resources better for giving her more nourishment, taking her to hospitals comfortably, getting her clothes to keep her warm, like that. (Savitri, caregiving adopted mother)

Yet, given their economic conditions, none of these four caregivers could contemplate providing their loved one with anti-retroviral treatment, and hence medical intervention comprised good nutrition, a healthy lifestyle and treatment for opportunistic infections. Realising this, caregivers felt that though they were doing their best within their circumstances, it was not enough.

Doctors say that though this illness has no cure, it can be stalled by taking some very expensive medicines (anti-retrovirals)—it seems that costs about 1,000–2,000 rupees a day. But what to do—that is completely beyond my means. I always feel bad about that—this facility exists but we cannot avail of it because we are poor. So the effort to help him is not complete in that sense, even though I am doing whatever is in my capacity—that is my only regret. (Rohit, caregiving brother)

However, caregivers from homes with modest resources did not believe that seeking assistance from the social network was a solution to the economic condition. While people from the social network were generally from the same social strata as they were and had their own concerns, caregivers also realised that since the HIV infection has a long-drawn out course and poses many financial demands, they cannot constantly depend on the social network for help but need to manage independently as much as possible.

Asking others for money to help us is not really a good idea. First of all, borrowing is not good—it is embarrassing. And then on top of that, later one has to repay. And in this illness, it continues for so long and just gets worse that how long can one borrow? Then, those special medicines (anti-retrovirals) cost the earth so one cannot think of borrowing that kind of amount. And from whom to borrow—our friends and acquaintances are as poor as us, they have their own problems. So just manage on one's own as far as possible. Only in extreme circumstances when there is no way out, then we can think of asking others—that is what we three decided. (Savitri, caregiving adopted mother)

This decision eliminated the option of seeking anti-retroviral treatment, since resources for this were unavailable. Nonetheless, caregivers were resigned to this as they were uncomfortable with the idea of having to ask others and later arrange for repayment. They sought to manage as much as possible on their own and anticipated seeking financial help only for pressing needs that could not be postponed or ignored.

The fifth caregiver, an upper-income group doctor who was looking after his positive father and brother, wished to provide them with the best treatment available. However, he perceived his resources as limited, given the expensive nature of the treatment, the length of time involved and the number of family members requiring it. Having to provide care to more than one HIV-positive person at the same time, for extended periods and at exorbitant costs, was proving to be a source of considerable anxiety. The caregiver was very troubled that under the circumstances, his resources would not permit him to provide the best care to his family members. He also anticipated the possibility of having to choose between the two infected family members in order to make decisions about the allocation of family resources, and this was described as a stressful dilemma for him.

Because there are two people (father and brother) infected in the house, the demands on me are much higher than if there had been just one. When they fall sick, it will be tough. We will have to divide our attention between both of them. Then there will be the financial costs—things are expensive in this illness, and one will have to plan for that. What I feel is that basically, I will give both of them an equal chance. Of course, my dad is 68 years old and so we will have to see whether he can tolerate the treatment or not. If he can, then I would like to give him the benefit, though if he refuses, I will not force him. With my brother, he is young and so if he cannot tolerate, I will find an alternative, and if he refuses, I will force him. Finally, if I have to choose between them, I will opt for my brother definitely, because he is younger and he has his whole life ahead of him. I think that that would be the right thing to do, though I would definitely consult other doctors before deciding. (Arvind, caregiving son and brother)

When HIV arises as a result of, and in addition to, an existing chronic health condition, it extends the caregiving role. One caregiver was looking after her thalassemic adolescent son, whose HIV infection was the result of transfusions with untested, contaminated blood. The caregiving mother described how she and her husband (who shared the caregiver role with her) experienced extensions of, and additions to, their current caregiving and other roles. Not only had they been already performing the caregiving role over a long period of time, but HIV with its attendant implications of stigma, death, debilitation and possible transmission, added to their problems. The hereditary link in the transmission of thalassemia caused them to feel responsible for their son's predicament and added to their distress.

First, he (son) had the thalassemia and for that, basically we (husband and I) had to see to his transfusions and injections. We had to be very regular, very vigilant about this—any carelessness could be problematic. And the entire day would go in visiting the hospital so we had to manage the time— my husband would take him to the hospital in the morning while I prepared breakfast and lunch and sent the other child to school—then I would go the hospital and my husband would go to work. We also used to feel bad to see him suffer— especially since he got it because of us. But HIV has made it all worse. We feel even more guilty, because he is suffering for no fault of his own, and the suffering is so much more than earlier. He has nothing to look forward to in his life. On top of it, we have to maintain great secrecy, unlike with thalassemia where we could share our troubles with others. He falls ill off and on, so we have to follow up treatment more often, so more running around, more time constraints and physical stress. His health is also deteriorating, so more care is needed. We have to be cautious about blood spillages, that too when nose bleeds are so common in thalassemics in the summer months. So a free mind is not there, as it had been in the past. (Sukanya, caregiving mother)

The woman reported acute health problems, arising from the prolonged physical strain of providing care and performing other domestic roles. However, she never allowed her ill-health to come in the way of doing her best for her son. On the contrary, she would ignore her own condition to see to his needs.

> I am completely exhausted. We (husband and I) have been looking after him for a long time and in last two years, his condition is worsening. Managing his treatment and his illness as well as the house and work, just the two of us have to do it—it is very tiring, we usually never get a chance to just sit and relax. I feel sleepy all the time, my body is tired. I get fever very often, feel weak all the time. But whatever it is, I never let it interfere with looking after him. Like, for his thalassemia, the doctor had told us in the beginning that tea is good for him, to prevent the iron from accumulating. So from that time, I have it in my mind that he should have tea. So no matter how tired I am, no matter what time of day or night it is, if he asks for tea, I get up and give him tea. If I am not well, he tells me, 'Mummy, don't bother', but I still do it. I feel that as much as I do for him, there is always a lot left to do. (Sukanya, caregiving mother)

Problems with physical health were similarly reported by two elderly caregivers, but these were never allowed to hamper role performance.

> I have all kinds of problems—heart, blood pressure/BP, arthritis. Seeing to all these things—the house, cooking, washing clothes, cleaning vessels, and then on top of it, seeing his (son's) condition and looking after him, makes me more sick. When he was in hospital (prior to diagnosis), it was even worse because then I had to run around a lot. Even coming here (to NGO C which is located on the outskirts of the city) is really exhausting for me, after completing all the housework. But I just do it all because I know that finally, if I put in the effort, it will help him. So I never let anything interfere. (Anita, caregiving mother)

The healthcare system was perceived as the creator of their difficult family situation by two caregivers. Here, care receivers

were infected by contaminated blood and IV (intravenous) equipment due to callousness on the part of health service organisations,
and this precipitated anger in their caregivers. One caregiver, who
was a doctor, believed that this experience was part and parcel of
the rural health setting, where no standards are maintained.

> He (father) had malaria when he was at the native place. See,
> rural places, they have a practice of giving everything intrave-
> nously. The set-up was a nursing home, and in small towns,
> they are not careful about equipment, so there must have been
> some contamination. (Arvind, caregiving son and brother)

For the other caregiver, whose thalassemic son received transfusions from a public hospital known for its programme on thalassemia (Hospital E), the healthcare system was no longer seen as
a reliable source of care and treatment. At the same time, not
only did the limited treatment options available restrict the search
for an alternative, but finding an alternative was also seen as
futile since the damage had already been done.

> They (Hospital E staff) did not take care, they did not test
> the blood and so this happened. Because there is no proper
> information in India, it is bound to happen. Why has it (HIV)
> not spread so much in other places as it has in India? Be-
> cause they take care over there and here they do not bother.
> So now we have got it in our house. But what to do? There
> are such few hospitals helping out thalassemics and espe-
> cially those with HIV, that we have to go there only (Hospi-
> tal E). I feel bad but then I feel, forget it, what has happened
> one should not think about. (Sukanya, caregiving mother)

Beyond this, the healthcare system's role in the caregiving trajectory was seen as mixed: facilitating care at times and hinder-
ing it at others. The public health system was looked at negatively, while the voluntary sector was seen as an important con-
tributor to the caregiving process. The role of private health services was not clearly demarcated.

Though two caregivers indicated that on receipt of the positive
diagnosis their care receivers' treatment was transferred from the
private hospitals where they were seeking care, to a specific public

hospital known to handle such cases (Hospital A), caregivers were far from satisfied with their experiences here. Since Hospital A was located at one end of the city, accessing treatment from there entailed high indirect costs in terms of travel expense, travel time and waiting time, that caregivers could ill afford because of economic factors and other role demands. Moreover, as the infection advanced, caregivers found travelling to Hospital A physically strenuous for themselves and their care receivers.

Besides the two caregivers whose care receivers' treatment was relocated to Hospital A following the diagnosis of HIV, two other caregivers continued accessing care from the public hospitals that they had been visiting prior to diagnosis (Hospitals A, C, E, F and G).

All four caregivers maintained that the indifference on the part of the staff of these centres made them feel unsure as to whether they (the caregivers) knew enough about the infection and whether they were performing their caregiving role properly, besides causing them to feel alone in their struggle. According to the caregivers, treatment centres lacked counselling facilities that provided information about the HIV infection and its demands, as well as emotional and other forms of support which would help them in their role performance. As a result, positive people, their caregivers and their families were left to grapple with the situation on their own, in circumstances of stigma and isolation. Participants opined that hospital staff should spend time with them, explaining the infection and its course, indicating appropriate care strategies, suggesting solutions and alternatives to problems, and supporting them emotionally. This would help them feel more confident about the care they were providing, while promoting feelings of connectedness.

In the beginning, we (husband and I) did not know anything about the infection. The staff of Hospital E did not really explain anything to us. So based on our understanding, we used to wash his (son's) clothes separately and keep his glass, plate and cutlery separately. And if he had a temperature, we would be very scared to sit near him. But as we learnt from the experiences of other families, our fears dissipated, and we stopped keeping his things separately, or washing his clothes separately. We became much freer. But I feel that the doctors and nurses should have informed us, they should have counselled us—after all, this illness is such that there is so much of fear, so much of misunderstanding and one cannot even speak openly about it to anyone, so one is just trying to manage alone without knowing if it is right or wrong. I feel that some support is important. (Sukanya, caregiving mother)

The dissatisfaction of all four caregivers over the frequent lack of availability of medicines and of operational diagnostic facilities in the public-sector hospitals was apparent. Except for the caregiver whose care receiver was receiving assistance from NGO D, the others had to arrange for these elsewhere, usually on a payment basis.

We were told to go to Hospital A for treatment after he (brother) was diagnosed. But over there, though medicines are supposed to be given free in the dispensary, sometimes they would not be available. Then we had to buy them privately and this would be expensive for us. So you go there expecting certain things, but you come away disappointed. (Rohit, caregiving brother)

The later transfer of two care receivers to a residential facility run by a voluntary organisation (NGO C, described in Chapter 4) solved many of the caregivers' problems, since all the needs of the care receiver, including food, treatment, medicines and lodging, were taken care of in time and without any charges.

For three caregivers, then, the voluntary sector was seen as an important facilitator of their caregiving role. Though neither of the agencies had programmes specifically catering to the needs of caregivers, the services that they provided for the care receiver alleviated the burden on the caregiver, sparing them the task of having to fulfil those needs.

NGO C has helped me out a lot. They do not have any specific service for family members. But because they look after the patients so well and take care of all their needs like their medicines, food, check-ups, everything, that too without charging, our work becomes automatically less. Like when he (son) was in hospital, we still had to be present over there to see to his needs, but here (NGO C), it is not so.

Once the person is admitted here, everything is seen to by the staff. (Anita, caregiving mother)

Indeed, as described above, for two caregivers, admission of their seropositive family member to the residential facility (NGO C) was a respite from having to execute caregiving tasks and from resource-related difficulties, though NGO C was not designed with caregivers in mind, nor had the caregivers admitted their care receivers there with the objective of gaining respite. The admission of care receivers to the residential facility was done as a stop-gap arrangement, taken because of the fear that their severe TB would be transmitted to young children in the home. While caregivers felt disturbed that they were not personally looking after their loved one, they were happy that the care receiver was receiving good and timely care, which helped them in their objective of helping him recover and prolonging his life. The respite that they received from executing caregiving tasks and the free service were added bonuses.

We (wife and I) decided to admit him (brother) here (NGO C) because of the TB—we were afraid that our children would catch the infection because the house is small—we all stay in the same room. I wanted to look after him at home itself, but for that, you need a big house. So the next best thing was for him to be here (at NGO C) till his TB subsides. Over here, the services are really good—the sisters (nuns in charge) take a lot of care. They check on the patients two, three times a day. If there is an emergency, ward members only need to call them and they come. They are not afraid to touch the patients, or to talk to them, and comfort them. Attention is really personalised. A doctor attends. Medicines are given on time, health status is monitored. Food is given on time and it is nutritious. So the whole set-up is geared to helping patients get better. We can call up and check how our family member is, we can speak to them too. If required, sisters call us up, and inform us how they are. Basically, we know that our family member is in good hands, and we need not worry at all. This location is also good—clean air, green, patients can walk about, they can pass their time with the TV and with the other patients. Though I would

have preferred to have looked after him myself at home, yet
this is a break from having to run around so much. (Rohit,
caregiving brother)

Nonetheless, caregivers and family members visited the positive person at the residential facility, bringing favourite foods,
toiletries, clothes and other items that had been requested for.
Family members spent time with the ill person, providing emotional support. They also monitored health status and progress by
conferring with the NGO C staff. If family members were unable
to visit every 2–3 days, they kept in touch with the staff via the
telephone in order to apprise themselves of their loved one's
progress. Staff members would also contact them telephonically,
if required. Family members continued to see themselves as responsible for their relative's well being.

Even though he (son) is here (NGO C) and the care is excellent, we keep track of his situation. After all, he is ours. I
visit him every 2–3 days, bring whatever he wants to eat.
Usually, I spend the whole day here when I come. The sisters
tell me about his health or I ask them. My daughter-in-law
rings them up regularly to find out how he is progressing—
even though she is so resentful of the whole situation, finally, it is our responsibility and she knows that. (Anita,
caregiving mother)

Caregivers appeared to be aware of the constraints voluntary
agencies faced in service delivery, such as limited resources and
high demand, and hence did not comment negatively about the
non-availability of anti-retroviral treatments here, though they
knew how important these were in stalling the progress of the
infection. On the contrary, they appreciated whatever they got,
realising that they were among a privileged few who benefited
from the voluntary sector and that the support they got was indispensable in facilitating better caregiving for them and longer survival for their care receivers.

They (NGO D staff) have to help so many people with basic
things—and that itself must be working out to a lot so how
can they give such expensive treatment? In fact, we are

lucky to get their help—not everyone does. I have met so many patients in the hospitals and none of them are getting this help. And as I told you, we are poor, so their assistance means a lot to us. (Savitri, caregiving adopted mother)

The caregiving doctor reported that his professional background helped him in his caregiving role. While he availed of the services of a private medical practitioner with considerable experience and expertise in the field of HIV/AIDS in order to get specialised service, his medical skills helped him to participate actively in the intervention process. Thus, not only did he get quality treatment for his care receivers, but because of his background, he could clearly comprehend the unfolding of the illness trajectory and appreciate the treatments required at specific times and for specific problems. He also received emotional support and moral courage from the doctor, which eased his anxiety.

... being a doctor has helped as I can cope better and deal with the situation appropriately. At one level, I take this illness as any other illness and I proceed as I normally would. The sense of responsibility is of course greater because they (father and brother) are my family members, and there are greater expectations of me. My doctor friends have put me in touch with a good physician who has been very supportive. He has helped me plan ahead, reassured me. Then (because of my background) I can understand the illness, the treatment, and so on ... what to expect, what to do, how to go about things. (Arvind, caregiving son and brother)

That the caregiving role and the constraints that contextualised it posed an undeniable burden for all the caregivers was quite visible. However, though the caregivers acknowledged their strain, there was no doubt in their mind that this strain was well worth it, since it was helping them achieve their objective of prolonging their loved one's life. They were happy that their efforts were helping their care receiver to live longer.

Yes, it is difficult for me. He (son) needs a lot of care when he is very ill and with my health problems, the resource problems, my daughter-in-law's attitude, my household tasks, it is very tough. But I don't mind because I want him to live—so no matter how strenuous I find it, I will not let that come in my way. I will just carry on because that will finally help him. (Anita, caregiving mother)

Indeed, caregivers stated that it was their intense motivation to save their family member's life that gave them the strength to cope and carry on, despite the various challenges they faced.

Whatever it is, we (husband and I) want him (son) to live. And I feel that that wish is what gives us our strength to go on. Because we feel that nothing we do is enough for him, there is always a lot left to do. So though we are very tired, looking after him for such a long time, we can still keep doing because we want to extend his life. (Sukanya, caregiving mother)

Though caregivers reported that they never expected any kind of reciprocity from their care receiver and that their provision of care did not depend on this, it was clear that all of them valued and cherished the care receiver's concern and appreciation. While caregivers' determination to save the life of their care receiving family member ensured that they would have provided care regardless of the latter's reaction, caregivers indicated that the feedback of the care receiver was seen as making their efforts all the more worthwhile. The bond between the caregiver and the care receiver deepened as a result.

Looking after him (son) has brought us closer. He knows that if it were not for me, no one would have bothered about him so much. He can see how his sister-in-law is. And when he tells me so, when he speaks out his appreciation, then I feel even more protective towards him ... because I feel he understands what it means to me to care for him ... and as a result, we relate to each other better. (Anita, caregiving mother)

Having seen their caregiving role as a fight against an early death, the passing away of a care receiver was seen as a personal failure by a caregiver. The latter believed that she had been unsuccessful in her role and could not forgive herself. Feelings of reproach hindered coming to terms with the loss and achieving closure on the experience, while also marring her earlier sense of satisfaction that arose from having undertaken such an arduous task.

> I did my best for her (adopted daughter), I thought I could make her live for a longer time but I failed. I feel that I went wrong somewhere and that is why this happened. When I think a lot about it, it seems unforgivable. And then I feel that may be I should have done more. So whatever satisfaction I got from looking after her dissipated with her death. (Savitri, caregiving adopted mother)

6

PRESERVING FAMILY AND LEARNING WHOM TO COUNT ON

There were five participants in the study who were seropositive women and who had been caregivers for their seropositive husbands. At the time of data collection, these women, whose ages ranged from 27–38 years, were widowed. All of them, except one, lived in neolocal residences with their children. Following the death of her husband, one woman had returned to her natal home after a property dispute with her in-laws. All the women were earning for their families, though four were mildly symptomatic. For all the women, support came from their natal families, despite the geographical distance in three cases. Adolescent children were assisting their mother in one case (see Table 6.1).

All the women stated that their seropositive status was because of their husbands. However, only four of them knew that their husbands had become infected through pre-marital and/or extra-marital multipartner sex. One woman said that though she believed that she had got the infection from her husband since he had fallen ill and passed away before her, she had no idea how he had acquired it. During the caregiving trajectory, all the women were asymptomatic.

The women's experiences revolved around two themes: preserving family and learning whom to count on.

PRESERVING FAMILY

Preserving family extended over two phases in the illness trajectory. During the lifetime of their husbands, women perceived their

Table 6.1

Profile of seropositive caregiving wives

Participant	Age	Education	Occupation	Marital status/No. of children	Present health status (symptom level)	Care receiver	Reported mode of infection	Informal support system/ caregiver	Co-residence/ proximity with caregiver/informal support system	HH income at the time of data collection (per month)
1	33	4th	Self-employed	Widowed/3	Asymptomatic	Deceased husband	Sexual (from husband)	Natal family	Natal family in native village 4–5 hours from Mumbai	600
2	36	10th	Permanent employee in a public hospital	Widowed/1	Mild	Deceased husband	Sexual (from husband)	Natal family	Natal family in neighbouring suburb	2,000
3	38	–	Piece rate temporary worker	Widowed/2	Mild	Deceased husband	Sexual (from husband)	Natal family	Natal family in native village in North India	850
4	30	–	Piece rate temporary worker	Widowed/2	Mild	Deceased husband	Sexual (from husband)	Natal family and children	Natal family in native village in North India; Co-residence with children	500 to 700
5	27	10th	Self-employed	Widowed/1	Mild	Deceased husband	Sexual (from husband)	Natal family	Lives with natal family following death of husband	3,250

role to be an attempt to extend the life of the husband, so that the family could remain intact, the children could benefit from the presence of both the parents and the women were spared the pains and problems of widowhood and single parenthood. It also meant helping husbands recover to their asymptomatic stage so that they could resume their earner roles, thereby restoring the family economy.

Following the death of the husbands, preserving the family related to women's endeavours to maintain their own health so that they could survive long enough to rear their children into adulthood, by which time the latter would be capable of standing on their own feet. According to the women, this was very important because the presence of a biological parent till that time was very critical, since the parent–child bond was irreplaceable during the formative years. Preserving family was also an attempt to provide the children with as happy a family life as possible, by protecting them from material deprivation and emotional distress, notwithstanding the loss of their fathers.

For four wives, equating caregiving as preserving the family began when wives heard the seropositive diagnosis. Upto that time, though the husbands had been falling ill periodically, the illness was seen as a passing phase, and caregiving was perceived as looking after the needs of the husbands that arose as a result of illness.

> Well, he (husband) was falling ill off and on for quite some time—that time, I just thought it would pass off and I would do whatever was required—like what one does normally when a family member is ill. But when I got to know about this AIDS illness and that it had no cure, then I knew that it was different ... it was like I had to not just see to his needs and medicines, but I had to help him to live so that my child could have a full life. (Rima)

The knowledge of the seropositive diagnosis made wives realise that they could lose their husbands and that that would have disastrous implications for themselves and their children. Realising the significance of their husbands' survival for the future of their children and for their own social status in a patriarchal society, the women began to perceive their role as ensuring the survival of their families.

I wanted him (husband) to live ... I only felt that if he got well it would be good for all of us, we would be a complete family, the children would have their father, no one would call me a widow, both of us would be able to earn and we would all be happy. But if he died, then the children and I would both suffer a lot ... children's future would be jeopardised and people would treat me badly because you know how widows are looked at ... so I did my best ... the diagnosis made me feel that I was not just looking after his health, no, it was more than that, I was saving the family. (Diya)

The fatal outcome associated with a positive diagnosis was found to greatly disturb wives, but they put aside their feelings so that they could channelise all their energies into prolonging their husband's life. However, they reported that putting aside their feelings did not amount to coming to terms with them, instead they were aware of a constant sense of sadness that pervaded their existence.

When I heard his (husband's) diagnosis, understood what it meant, I felt that the world had collapsed around me ... but if I gave in, if I got overwhelmed by my feelings, then we would be nowhere because I would be too upset to help him or to save my family. So I just stopped myself from thinking about it and went about my work—but I was always sad, always depressed, I just ignored it all for my children's sake. (Falguni)

The fifth woman underwent testing as a part of antenatal care for her second pregnancy. When she was found to be HIV-positive, her husband too was tested and found infected. Both of them were asymptomatic at the time. The woman's child was found to be positive at birth and passed away soon afterwards. Symptoms started first in the husband and when this began, the woman put in every effort to save her husband's life for herself and for her elder child.

Though wives themselves were positive, they were not concerned about their own health status since they were asymptomatic. They believed that they were in good health and would remain so for many years to come. Their attention was riveted on getting their husbands back to an asymptomatic/mildly symptomatic stage so that they could lead an active life.

> I did not bother about myself because I was in good health anyway. I was only concerned about him (husband) and getting him back to normal. That was important for us. (Urvashi)

The adoption of this orientation resulted in women completely forgetting about themselves. For example, four women knew that their husbands had acquired HIV as a result of lifestyles of drinking, gambling and multipartner pre-marital/extra-marital sex. These lifestyles, which had been present prior to and continued during marriage, were responsible for marital strife and a drain on family resources. Women, who had from the time of marriage harboured anger towards their husbands for their habits, found their negative feelings exacerbated after they heard the seropositive diagnosis. They were very disturbed when they realised the costs of their husbands' actions, but none of them communicated their feelings to their husbands. They believed that the latter were suffering enough from the knowledge of the diagnosis and from opportunistic infections. Chiding them was seen as intensifying their emotional distress, which would be detrimental to their speedy recovery. None of the women, therefore, allowed their feelings to influence the caregiving process. In spite of their anger, they provided the best possible care so that their husbands could improve.

> Yes, he (husband) created a lot of problems for us. From the time of marriage, he would drink, disappear for 2–3 days, spend a lot of money and I used to be very angry but it was of no use, he would not listen. Now because of his behaviour only he got AIDS, and my daughter and I have had to suffer. But I never once let my anger affect my caregiving. I never said anything to him—why upset him more when he is already suffering? I just put it all aside and cared for him with a clean and willing heart—I did my best, leaving no stone unturned ... because otherwise, if I had been angry and all that, then maybe the care would have not been good enough and he would not survive. (Rima)

Women's descriptions of the care they provided highlight the effort they made.

Initially, the illness episodes were of a temporary nature and they were not so severe, so I had essentially to supervise his (husband's) treatment and care—accompany him to the doctor, see that he took his medicines, give him his food on time and so on. But as he got more and more ill, my tasks also increased. I had to do more and more for him. There were times when he was too weak to move, and I used to carry him to the bathroom and the toilet. I used to give him a bath and keep him clean, at home and in the hospital. I used to take him to the hospital for his treatment, and sometimes when he was too weak to go by public transport, I used to arrange for a private taxi. Sometimes, if he did not have to meet the doctor, I would go on my own for the medicines. Making sure that he ate properly was a priority. I never stinted on food, even though I had to borrow. And whatever he asked for, I would get for him. When he was in the last stages, he could not eat any solid foods, and because of the burning in his throat, he preferred to drink cold drinks, so I would keep cold drinks for him. When people would visit and ask what they should get for him, I would request them to bring cold drinks only. In the last three months, I had to do everything for him—I had to even feed him. When he was in hospital, I remained with him day and night. I always reassured him too. After he got to know he was HIV positive, he was so depressed, so hopeless, and I would always keep his spirits up … I always told him that I would never leave him and that he should not worry on that account … I would do things for him without him having to ask me. There were times when even at home, I would never sleep the whole night seeing to him … my entire attention and life revolved around him. I never use to bother about myself at that time. I felt that whatever happens to me let it happen, but *aapla jhevda hota to paryant aapan karyacha seva tyachi* (as much as I can do, I must do for him) … so that he can live. (Rima)

Women were essentially sole caregivers, supported in their roles by their natal families and by voluntary organisations. With this support, they took responsibility for caregiving and executed all caregiving tasks. As the quote above describes, the content of care varied with the severity of the infection. Mild episodes called for assistance with visits to doctors/healthcare centres, administering and supervising medicines, and monitoring health status. These tasks were expanded to include hands-on physical care and assistance with bodily functions during bouts of severe illness and incapacitation. Emotional care and good nutrition were provided throughout.

Hospitalisation influenced the caregiving process. Three wives reported that their husbands had undergone hospitalisation in public hospitals in the post-diagnosis phase, sometimes on more than one occasion and in more than one public hospital. In Hospitals A and I, though staff were supportive in orientation, they generally provided limited assistance to in-patients, and expected family members to be present to fulfil patient needs. Women's caregiving tasks continued during this time. Where illness was not so severe, wives could afford to take breaks to perform other roles and responsibilities, especially child care. However, when the illness was severe, wives had no choice but to be physically present in the hospital all the time to look after their husbands. This meant making appropriate arrangements for the execution of their other roles and responsibilities (especially child care) that they had to forego to accommodate caregiving in the hospital.

He (husband) was admitted in hospital 2–3 times. But it is not a break from seeing to him or anything. In the beginning, when he was not so ill, then of course, I could leave him there and do my other work, see to ____ (child), keep him there by himself at night—because his condition was such that he was fairly independent, go to the bathroom on his own, move about ... but later in the last three months when he was at Hospital A, his condition was so bad that he was completely bed-ridden and these hospitals will not take care of all your needs, they expect a family person to be there. So I had to be there all the time. I left ____ (child) with my sister-in-law and if I had to meet her, then I would ask my brothers to be with him and then I could go. Or if I had to contact the NGO D people, then I would phone them or ask my sister-in-law to sit with him (husband) while I

went to meet them. So 24 hours, someone was needed because everything of his was being taken care of on the bed
only, so someone had to be there. (Rima)

In other hospitals (G and H), the fear of transmission and stigma
associated with the infection caused the staff to not only completely neglect in-patients, but to publicly demean them, and hence
families had no choice but to cease taking treatment from these
hospitals and turn to others like Hospitals A and I.

In Hospital G (a public hospital), when he (husband) was
admitted, the staff told everyone in the ward that he had
AIDS, and so everyone began to isolate him and speak about
him. He got so upset that in the night, he wore someone
else's clothes and came away. We never went back to Hospital G again. (Urvashi)

Caregiving, especially during severe illness episodes and
hospitalisation, put a lot of strain on the women, and given the
long-drawn nature of the HIV infection, this continued for an extended period of time.

While four women lived in nuclear households, one woman
lived with her in-laws. Withdrawal of support from the in-laws
following knowledge of the diagnosis implied that the woman
had to manage on her own, though she continued to live in the
in-law household. Thus, as a result of their husband's illness,
women had to take charge of their families. Regarding the availability of economic resources for family survival, during mild episodes husbands were able to maintain their earner role, though
being unwell and sometimes requiring rest or hospitalisation entailed a few days of absence for which salary cuts were made,
depending on the nature of the job. One husband, employed as a
temporary daily wage earner, lost his job because of his HIV status and began to serve liquor in his home in order to earn a
living. Only one woman was employed, being involved in home-
based piece rate part time work that supplemented her husband's
income. During this period, then, women had a more or less steady
income to rely on.

However, when illness severity grew, not only did the concomitant increase in caregiving responsibilities leave the earning

wife with no time for her paid work, but all the husbands' physical conditions hindered them from working. Nonetheless, two husbands in permanent posts in government hospitals received their salary as long as they had leave to their credit, while one man with his own business of serving liquor was able to continue with it since he was operating out of his home. Women in the rest of the families had to arrange for resources, as did women in the three preceding families when their husbands' incomes stopped.

> Initially when he (husband) used to fall ill, it was only for a few days and it was very mild, so there was no real problem about working—he would maybe take a day or two off, maximum a week, and then get back to work. So money was coming into the house. But when his condition became severe, he was in the hospital for three months—I had to be with him all the time, so I also could not earn. That time, my source of income was the rent from the two rooms we own. (Falguni)

Since caregiving and family responsibilities precluded four women from taking up, and one woman from continuing with, paid employment outside the home, their finances came from various sources—one woman took up the running of her husband's alcohol business; another dipped into her savings; two took loans; and one received some income from the renting of two rooms that she owned.

None of the four women who owned property, or whose husbands owned property, contemplated selling it off at this juncture, since they considered this to be important assets to retain for their children's future.

As a result of the changes in the earning patterns and income sources of the family and the expenses associated with HIV-related treatment, economic drain and material deprivation set into the families.

> For one year, I was managing with my savings of Rs 7,000 so we had to cut down on things ... like we would eat nutritious food but nothing fancy, we could not go out much like for outings for the children ... so many things we had been getting earlier we had to do without. (Sona)

Yet, medical, material and financial support from NGOs and from natal families helped the women out to some extent, cushioning the intensity of the economic impact. While four women obtained support from NGO D and one got medical assistance from NGO A, four women received financial/material support from their natal families. One woman's natal family was too poor to help her out materially and financially.

When he (husband) was very ill and admitted to Hospital K (a public hospital), I informed my people in the village (in North India) about it. They sent my sister's husband to help me out. They sent Rs 8,000 with him for me. And he stayed with us for three months looking after the children while I was in hospital with my husband. At that time, he was working also and whatever he earned, he would spend on the children ... then, at Hospital A, the staff put me in touch with NGO D and they helped us out with food, medicines, children's education. All this helped us to manage because otherwise, we only had the rent from the rooms. (Falguni)

Resource allocation within the household always favoured the men, followed by the children. Women ensured that men got the best that they could provide with their resources in terms of nutrition and treatment for opportunistic infections, believing that this was indispensable for saving their husband's life. Women put themselves last, though they were also positive and needed to take care of their health.

He (husband) always came first—for everything. Whatever money I had, I would always use it for him first, and then only think of my child and then me—so whatever I could afford, I would give him the best food, treatment, whatever, so that his life could be extended. About myself, I was not concerned as such. (Urvashi)

While working tirelessly for their husbands, however, women did not neglect their children. Children remained with the parents throughout the father's illness trajectory, except at times of hospitalisation when women's natal families looked after them. For one woman whose natal family lived in a native village in

North India, a male member of the family came and stayed with the children during this time, so that the wife could be with the husband in the hospital.

Besides ensuring that children's physical, material and, where applicable, educational needs were taken care of as best as possible, given the resources at their disposal, mothers sought to protect their children emotionally. Mothers would provide various explanations to young children, laced with hope and recovery, to answer their questions and allay their distress about their father's condition. Episodes of hospitalisation, which necessitated the mother's absence from the child, were similarly explained.

> When he (husband) was very ill, she (child) would observe how bad his condition was and she used to ask me, 'What is wrong with Papa, why is he sleeping so much, why does he not take me out like before?' So I would tell her that he is not well and he needs to take a lot of rest so that he can play with you and take you out. I would say that with this rest, he will be well and then we can all go out and enjoy ourselves. Things used to be quiet in the house also, so that would upset her mood too. I would spend time with her, playing with her or telling her amusing stories to distract her and cheer her up. When he was in the hospital, she was with my sister-in-law and when I would back home, I would tell her that your father is not well so I am with him, helping him to get well and when he is well, then we can all go out and play together. So she would say, 'OK, Mummy, you look after Papa and when he gets well, you bring him back'. (Rima)

The situation was more difficult to handle in one family where the adolescent son had initially picked up the father's diagnosis from the family's social network, and later informed his younger brother about it. Offspring, here, since they understood the terminal prognosis of HIV/AIDS, reacted with hopelessness, but the mother comforted them by referring to her attempt to stall the progress of the infection. In this way, the mother sought to build up hope in the children that the father would survive for some time.

> The news of his (husband's) diagnosis had spread in the locality where we were living at that time. And someone

told my elder son about it—so he got to know and told his brother too. They were old enough and they could understand what it meant so they were very disturbed and upset. They came to me and said, 'Papa is going to die and then we will be left alone to rot and die. How will we manage, who will bother about us? We will have to beg and live on the streets.' I comforted them by explaining how the illness took years to reach the end and if one took care, this could be stalled. And I told them how I was taking a lot of care of the father so that he could live and that way, things would be fine for us. So they did feel better but I guess at the back of their minds, they must have had some anxieties. After they spoke about their concerns to me, I always tried to maintain hope in them. (Sona)

Women did not seek any assistance with caregiving tasks from their children for two equally important reasons—the children's developmental stage and the fear of transmission of the virus in instances of hands-on physical care.

So focused were the women on their goal that they were not conscious of the strain it involved and of the implications this could have for their own health when they too were positive. They knew only that they had to save the lives of their husbands, at all costs. That they were positive and in need of care did not seem to matter much to them. It was obvious that throughout the caregiving trajectory, women put themselves last. Only in the post-death phase did women become conscious of their physical strain and fatigue.

I never considered my own life at that time. I was also having this illness but I never bothered about it. My thoughts were all for him (husband)—I just wanted to save his life and so I put everything aside. I did not bother about my sleep, my health. I just ran around a lot to get his treatment done, to get money, to see to him, my child and the house. It was tiring, but I did not bother—in fact, it never struck me then. I never thought of myself. And anyway, I had no time to think—I never stopped doing—I was all the time doing. I must have been tired but at that time it never struck me. How I never felt it, I don't know—it never occurred to me,

God only knows. After he died, then I realised how exhausted
I was and I wondered how I had managed so much. (Rima)

Upto a point of time during the unfolding of the infection, wives
maintained their belief that husbands could recover from severe
illness episodes. Since this did happen quite a few times over the
illness trajectory in three cases, wives in these instances grew
firmer in their belief. All the wives thus believed that preserving
their families was possible and worked towards this. However, at
a particular juncture, when severe illness did not show any signs
of abating, but on the contrary progressively worsened, women
realised that they would not able to save the lives of their husbands and that their dream of preserving their families would not
fructify. Women were then engulfed in grief and uncertainty. Coming to terms with these developments was not easy for the women,
since they had long nurtured their hopes for an intact family, but
the demands presented by their various roles and responsibilities
left them with little time to attend to their feelings. Putting aside
their emotional turmoil, women continued to care for their husbands and children, with a little more help from their natal families and NGOs. They sought to make the last days of their husbands' lives as comfortable as possible. This was spelt out in terms
of the provision of physically comfortable surroundings, the reduction of physical pain and discomfort, optimal satisfaction of as
many needs as possible, including emotional solace and the reassurance of being loved and valued. They also worked towards
maintaining optimism and hope in their children. Determined to
continue to do their best for their families, even at this stage,
women remained unaware of the strain they were undergoing.

When I first heard he (husband) had this AIDS, I was so
determined to help him survive and I worked very hard for
it—I was sure that he would because the doctors said that if
we looked after him properly, he could live for 15–20 years.
So that kept me going. But later he grew worse and there
was never any improvement, so after some time, I realised
that this was it, there was no going back at all ... I was so
upset when that happened, I can't tell you—so upset, so
defeated, so hopeless ... but what to do? I had to see to him
and the child anyway. I could not let my feelings overpower

me, otherwise who would do? And there was so much to do—look after him, see to the house, see to my daughter. So I had to carry on as before … I knew he had little time left so I tried to make him as comfortable as possible—attend to his needs, cheer him up, reassure him that I would be there for him. I was so caught up with it all that I never realised how much I was doing or how fatigued I felt. (Urvashi)

Throughout the caregiving trajectory, task-oriented as they were in dealing with the situation, women drew comfort from the presence of the natal family and NGOs, and from spiritual sources. According to them, the support of their natal families and of the staff of NGO A or D (as the case may have been), helped them to deal with many of the challenges that they faced, while also reassuring them that there were people they could turn to, if needed. The presence of these people provided the women with a sense of connectedness that facilitated their coping.

Because of these people (from NGO D) and my (natal) family, I could manage—they helped me deal with so many things. Like money, medicines, food, children's education, being with the children when I was with him (husband) in the hospital—these people only helped me, otherwise, how would I have managed? Because they were there with me, I felt that there is someone with me and that thought gave me courage. (Falguni)

It was common for the woman to adopt philosophical outlooks to explain their predicament. Referring to fate, dharma, *naseeb* and kismat helped women to accept their experiences.

What is in one's fate will happen. This AIDS was in my *naseeb*, so what to do? I had to live like that. (Sona)

Women also coped by ignoring their emotional turmoil. They did this because they felt that recognition of, and importance given to, feelings would overwhelm them to the extent of crippling their ability to function. Therefore, suppression of feelings became an important means of dealing with the situation.

I would ignore my feelings most of the time. If I allowed myself to get affected and just incapacitated with grief, then I would have just broken down, and who would have done so much for him (husband). (Rima)

Wives reported a sense of satisfaction in the knowledge that they had done their best. Not only did they put in every effort to preserve their families, but they carried out their spousal duty faithfully regardless of their husbands' earlier behaviour. It was important for them that they should not be found wanting in their role performance by others, and they knew that the care they provided allowed them to maintain their self-respect and the dignity of their natal family in society.

I am proud that I left aside nothing in caring for him (husband). Of course, he is my husband so I have to do it. Whether he treated me properly or not, it is a wife's duty to stick by the husband and so I did it. Otherwise, the world will say that since the husband is ill, she left him ... people will say that her parents did not bring her up properly. (Sona)

From their husbands, wives expected nothing but an acknowledgement of their contribution. This was perceived as more meaningful than any material offering. Therefore, the indifference of the husbands was one of the most painful parts of the caregiving trajectory. Husbands, whose lifestyles were responsible for acquiring the infection and passing it on to their wives, showed no feelings about their behaviour, nor did they demonstrate any concern towards their wives about their health status and the strain that caregiving and managing the family were causing. Appreciation for caregiving was not forthcoming either. Wives recognised and reacted to the indifference of their husbands, though they did not let their feelings affect the caregiving process. There were feelings of hurt that besides having infected them, the husbands displayed a lack of concern and of appreciation.

He (husband) was not bothered about me—because of him, I had got AIDS, I was in this position (of having to do so much and undergo so much of strain looking after him and the family), but he was not bothered at all. He would never even ask how I was, how I was managing. I was hurt, deeply hurt .... Sometimes I feel very disappointed that he had no appreciation for all that I did for him. But I still carried on, as before. (Sona)

It was only when they were nearing death that four husbands expressed appreciation and concern. Three of them did so directly to their wives, while one wife overheard her husband describe his positive feedback to a friend. The husbands acknowledged that the wives had gone out of their way to look after them, when even their own families of origin had rejected them. They were also concerned that the wives should look after themselves. Wives were found to cherish these expressions of appreciation and sensitivity. They felt that their commitment to the care of their husbands was rewarded.

Even though his (husband's) appreciation came only at the end, it meant a lot to me. I had stood by him throughout, put up with all his ways. What his own family was not willing to do, I did. So naturally, that he appreciated it made me feel that all my sacrifice and care were all worth it. If he had never said it, I would have felt that I had made no difference, that I did not matter to him. (Urvashi)

Following the death of their husbands, when the caregiving role ceased, women became conscious of their physical strain and fatigue. Seeing how tired they were and thinking back over all they had done, women were taken aback by their own performance and reported in retrospect that they had no idea how they had managed multiple demanding tasks over an extended period of time. They believed that their single-minded focus of extending their husband's life and preserving their family propelled them to do so. It was during the post-death phase that women realised that they needed to take care of themselves, in order to stall the progress of the infection and prolong their lives so that they could care for their children and rear them into adulthood. Thus, the fact that they themselves were care receivers sunk in only at this stage.

After he (husband) died then I began to feel so tired, so exhausted—I realised that I had lost weight, felt weak. I realised then that I had been so caught up in looking after him that I had not even paid attention to myself. But I had to look after myself now because I was also positive and I was all my children had, so I had to look after myself for them. I guess after he died, there was so much less to do that I had the time to think, to sit, to just do nothing, so all these thoughts dawned on me. The fatigue must have been there all along since I had so much of running around and tension when he was ill, but I was not aware of it as such. Seeing to him and the children was my priority and my life revolved around this, so I had no time to consider myself. Now I sometimes wonder how I did all that, that too by myself ... I had to see to him and the children, the house and the business (the couple served liquor in their home in order to earn), all by myself. Children are small and he was totally on bed—everything on bed at the end, he was like a child ... I had to feed him, give him the bedpan, urinal, bathe him. And the entire day, he wanted me to massage his feet. I used to be tired because I never would get sleep. Every night I would be awake the whole night, massaging his feet. No sleep at all. At 5 AM, I would get up, make chapatis and bhaji, and then wake up the children, get them ready and take them to school. Then come back, see to him, go to market, cook—by then, I had to bring the children back. In the afternoon, take them for tuitions. In the evening, we used to do the business—that we had to do, or how would we eat? So get the liquor, get the house ready ... I got no time for myself—sometimes, there was no time to even go to the bill meetings (the family was getting support from NGO D and bill meetings were organised by the NGO at which they reimbursed some expenses of the family and distributed rations). Even taking the children to school, or for tuitions, or going to the market, I would just run and come, not look here and there, so that I could come back soon and not leave him alone. But I guess I could do it because I had one goal—I wanted him to get well ... so I just pushed myself. Only later when he died, it occurred to me that I have to see to myself too because I have my children to see to and for their sake, I have to look after myself, so that I can be healthy and alive and look after them till they are big enough to manage on their own. (Diya)

In the post-death phase, four women who had earlier lived in nuclear families with neolocal residences continued with the arrangement, while one woman who had been living with her in-laws during the lifetime of her husband returned to her natal home (located in Mumbai) when, following a dispute with her in-laws over property division, the latter made her and her child leave their home.

Women staying independently spoke of their fears of living as widows with their children. They expressed insecurity about their safety, especially at night, as well as unhappiness that people around them would speak and think badly of them, since widows are not respected but viewed with suspicion in society. In order to protect themselves and their children, the women undertook various precautions. For example, the women stated that they were careful not to go out after sunset, because that caused people observing them to gossip about their movements. The women also never opened their doors after a certain time in the night, even if they heard a knock.

> Living alone with the children is a tension. Widows are always seen so negatively in our society and whatever they do, people always watch and comment, so one has to be so careful. Even if one is innocent, people attribute all sorts of bad things. At night, I get so tense that I cannot sleep. I am always worried who will come. So I sleep with an iron rod. What to do? I get scared. Generally, I close the door by 10 PM, and after that I never open it, even if I hear a knock. (Diya)

Despite their anxieties, returning to the natal family was not seen as an option for several reasons, even though natal families opened their doors to the women and their children. Three women's natal families lived away from Mumbai in the native village (two women's natal homes were in North India, while one woman's natal family belonged to a village located 4–5 hours from Mumbai). The women felt that relocating there would not only hamper their children's education, but also prevent them from getting good treatment, given the state of education and healthcare facilities in rural India. Moreover, the natal family of one of these women was too poor to support her materially/financially. Thus, even though she had relocated to the native village in North India when her husband's condition was severe, in order to get some family support and to transfer her husband's property to her children during his lifetime, she returned to Mumbai with her children after his death.

One woman, whose nuclear family lived in a neighbouring suburb, got a permanent post in the public hospital where her husband had been working (Hospital H). She was also given living quarters on the hospital premises, and hence wished to live there due to the proximity to her workplace. According to her, this would save her the trouble involved in commuting daily to work as well as in transferring her child to another school. It is important to mention here that though the positive status of this woman's husband had spread throughout his workplace and neighbourhood which were on the same premises (because of violations of ethical guidelines at the private nursing home where he had been tested), the wife's seropositive status had not spread. The wife's serostatus was not an issue for her appointment. She was neither asked her serostatus, nor recommended for testing by her employers. Co-workers did not raise the issue either.

During this time, women assumed the earner role. Not only did they see it as their responsibility to provide for their families, but since they were no longer performing the caregiving role, they were in a better position to take up paid employment. So, two women undertook piece rate home-based work, with one of them also receiving returns from the renting out of two rooms she owned, and one woman continued her husband's business of serving alcohol in her home. A fourth woman, as mentioned earlier, got a permanent job in the public hospital where her husband had been employed. The incomes of these women were supplemented by the nutritional, educational and medical support from NGO D, while one woman's adolescent son took up a job to assist the family. During this time, the women did not take any material or financial support from their natal families. Not only did they feel that they could manage with their income and NGO D's support, but they also felt that they had troubled their natal families sufficiently during the lifetime of their husbands and would be doing so once again when they fell severely ill.

Now that I have this job here (at Hospital H) and NGO D is also helping me out, I can manage comfortably. So I don't take anything from my people. Anyway, they did enough for me when he (husband) was alive and they will be the ones to look after me and ____ (child) later on, so why should I trouble them unnecessarily now when I can be independent? (Rima)

The woman who had returned to her natal family was economically independent because of the property she had inherited from her husband. This was a shop which she rented out and received returns on. In addition, her husband had been working as a permanent employee in a public hospital (Hospital F), and she had applied for a post over there on humanitarian grounds.

In the case of this woman as well another one, since their husbands had been employed in permanent posts in government hospitals, their jobs carried certain benefits which were given to their families in the event of their deaths. Thus, both these wives were entitled to their husband's benefits. However, one woman received nothing, since her husband had borrowed heavily against this amount for HIV-related treatment and household expenditures during the period when illness-related severity and the care it required prevented him and his wife from earning. Similarly, though the other woman received some money, she used most of what she got to pay back loans she had incurred for her husband's treatment and care, and for household expenses during the caregiving and severe illness trajectories, when neither she nor her husband was able to earn.

One woman became symptomatic soon after the death of her husband. Bouts of fever and diarrhoea alternated with periods of good health. During times of illness, the woman experienced considerable weakness which made movement difficult and warranted a lot of rest. With her natal family away in a North Indian village, it was her two adolescent sons who looked after her at these times, monitoring her health, supervising her medicines and accompanying her to the doctor if she was unable to go by herself. They also ran the house, completing cooking and cleaning chores. The woman expressed deep appreciation for the care provided by her sons. That her children put in so much effort to support her despite their young age touched her deeply. At the same time, she felt very guilty to have to subject them to such a situation, which was not only out of synchrony with their developmental stage, but which involved a role reversal. She felt that the presence of HIV/ AIDS in the family had forced her children to grow up before their time, depriving them of the normal milestones of adolescence. During illness episodes, the weakness that set in prevented the woman from continuing with her piece rate home-based work. She would resume this when she recovered.

> When I get fever and diarrhoea, then I feel very weak and I find it difficult to do much. My children look after me, then. After all, there is no one over here (in Mumbai). They make food, tea and give me. They wash the clothes, the vessels, come with me to the doctor. They are young but they do everything, they look after me very well ... show so much of concern. I feel bad ... which mother would not? To make the children do the work, to be looked after by them when they are so young ... they should not have any worries at this stage, but they cannot enjoy their youth. They are at the age when they still need my care but what is happening is opposite ... I feel sometimes that I have failed them and it troubles me a lot. (Sona)

Three other women developed symptoms some time after the deaths of their husbands. At the time of data collection, they were mildly symptomatic, with short-lived illness episodes that did not warrant much care. Nonetheless, for the woman living with her natal family, family members ensured that she rested and super-vised her treatment, accompanying her to the doctor.

> My symptoms are very mild but my (natal) family is very careful whenever I fall ill. They insist that I rest and take my medicines ... take me to the doctor. They take a lot of care. (Urvashi)

For the other two women, care was largely self-managed as one woman's natal family was too far away in a North Indian village, whereas the other woman whose natal family lived in the neighbouring suburb, felt that she had troubled them enough during her husband's illness and since her condition was very mild, she could manage on her own. These two women, then, would manage child care and household tasks, while also seeing to themselves, though depending on their physical condition they often suspended work for a few days.

> I manage on my own when I fall ill. After all, the children are young and my family is far away. Anyway, it is not very severe so I can manage without too many problems except that sometimes, if I feel too tired, I stop the work (piece rate work that she was engaged in) for a few days till I feel completely fine. (Falguni)

Within the constraints of their individual situations, women made sure that they maintained their health. They ate a nutritious diet, tried to avoid excessive physical exertion and tried to push away thoughts that made them tense and upset, though this was sometimes difficult, since they found themselves remembering the past, grieving for their husbands and worrying about the future. They also immediately sought medical intervention for their ailments and followed the treatment meticulously. Women believed that these activities were important so that they could live on for the welfare of their children.

> After he (husband) died, I knew that for the sake of the children, I had to live, I had to take care of myself. So I am very careful ... I eat well, try to rest, try to be happy and cheerful because they (staff of Hospital A) told me that if I get upset and depressed about this AIDS and its impact, it would not be good for me. If I get any illness, I at once take medicines, go to the doctor ... so like that, whatever I can do to maintain my health and keep well, I do. My children need me, so I have to do these things. (Falguni)

Looking after the needs of their children was also an ongoing activity. In the household with adolescent children, both of whom looked after the mother during illness episodes and the elder of whom was in paid employment to support the family, the mother, besides seeing to the material and physical needs of the children to the best of her ability, provided a lot of emotional support to them, helping them cope with their fears and anxieties. Children here were aware of their mother's diagnosis and anticipated losing her as they had the father. They were filled with uncertainty about the future, expressing misgivings about how they would manage on their own. The mother worked hard to allay their fears and boost their optimism and confidence, by highlighting their strengths, resources and capabilities and by pointing out the alternatives available.

> The children know what illness I have and they are scared because they have seen what happened to their father. So when I fall ill, they get very upset and cry. They say, 'We have no one else besides you so what will happen to us?' They live in that fear. So I always tell them that I will be there for sometime at least, since I am looking after myself, my condition was diagnosed in the beginning so I can take more care. I tell them that they are strong people who have been able to manage so much when I am ill and that that strength will help them survive, that in a city like Mumbai, there are always opportunities to earn a living ... that NGO D people are there ... that I will be leaving their father's property for them so they can go back to the village and live there where my (natal) family also is. I constantly try to calm them ... to instill confidence in them about the future. (Sona)

In the other four households, where children were younger, mothers took responsibility for all the children's needs, fulfilling them as well as their resources permitted. Besides physical and material needs, children would sometimes ask the whereabouts of the father and inquire when he would return, indicating that they experienced some void. Mothers, sensing the children's emotional distress, would attempt to reassure them through spiritual explanations, indicating that though the father was physically absent, he was psychologically present since he now lived with God and God's home permeated every part of the earth.

> Though she (child) is small, she realises that her father was there initially and now he is not there. Sometimes, it must be weighing on her mind, it must be puzzling her. She remembers how he used to play with her, take her out, so it must be upsetting her also. Once in a way, she asks me where he is, when he will come back. I tell her that he has gone to God's house and that even though we cannot see

him, he is around, he is thinking of us, he cares about us ...
he keeps a watch on us but we cannot see him because in
God's house, things are not visible to those who are not
there, but those who are in God's house, can see everything, can go wherever they want. That makes her feel better and she calms down. (Rima)

Overall, mothers stated that they made it a point not to inflict
any pain or sadness on their children—they ensured that their
interactions with their children conveyed love and happiness at
all times, so that the child could experience stability and comfort
in the midst of distress as well as have good memories to cherish
in the future.

I never do anything to hurt her (child) or make her sad.
After all, she has experienced so much of pain already at
such a tender age and I never want to add on to that, because I know that she anyway feels the loss of her father,
and if I hurt her then she will think that she has no one she
can rely on or turn to. So I always take care to make her feel
loved. Even if I have to correct her, I do it very gently and
affectionately. (Rima)

Notwithstanding their vigilance over, and attempts to maintain, their health, women harboured fears and uncertainties about
the future. That, finally, death was inevitable unless a cure for
the infection was found, troubled them. This was so because they
knew that it was possible that their conditions could worsen prior
to the discovery of a remedy, leaving the future of their children
in jeopardy.

I am doing my best to look after myself, but still one cannot
say about the future. The NGO D people said that so far,
there is no cure for the infection and that means that, in
case my condition worsens, there is no real hope. This
thought worries me a lot because then what will become of
my children? They will be bereft. (Falguni)

Planning ahead for the future of their children was, therefore,
seen as unavoidable. Relying on their natal family to help the

children out following their death was seen as indispensable, since the children would definitely require some support system, though the nature and degree of assistance required varied with the ages of the children. For the woman who had adolescent children, the role of the natal family was perceived as being more supervisory, whereas for the other four women with younger children, reloca- tion of the children to the natal family was imperative (and this had already happened in the case of the woman who moved back to the natal family after her husband's death).

> Finally, my mother, brother and sister will have to look after them (children). Even if I leave money and this house for them, they are too young to manage on their own. So that means that they will have to move to the native village where my people are ... they will have to stay with them. (Diya)

In the latter four instances, women expressed some misgiv- ings. They stated that though they believed completely in their natal families and vouched for their integrity, having their children looked after by others was not the same as doing so themselves. They believed that no matter how good the care others provide, a parent–child bond is irreplaceable. Women felt that by transferring the responsibility, they were failing as mothers, even though they had no doubts that their natal family would do a good job. They felt guilty about having to relinquish their maternal responsibilities when their offspring were still children, and were pained by the idea that they may be unable to see them grow into adulthood.

> My brother and sister-in-law will look after her (child) as if she is their own child—my sister-in-law is a gem of a person and my daughter is also very comfortable with her. They are so supportive, such nice people, that I have absolutely no reason to worry on that account. But still, I am the mother and somehow, there can be no replacement for that. I feel that my not being there for her means that she will always have some void, some emptiness in her life—so that makes me very disturbed. (Rima)

Three women, whose children were young and whose natal families knew their and their husbands' diagnoses, had spoken to their natal families about their future, though they acknowledged that knowing the supportive attitude of the natal family, they need not have done so—the natal family would do the needful anyway, without being requested. The natal families had willingly agreed to help out, with appeals to the women not to worry about the children's future. Women reported feeling reassured on this account though these positive feelings could not obliterate their misgivings and anxieties.

> My (natal) family has said that they will see to the children later on. Of course, I need not have asked them because knowing them, there was no doubt about it, they are completely dependable. In fact, they have told me that I should not be anxious on this account. But whatever it is, I feel bad that I will be not be there for my children and that I have to leave them to the care of others. (Falguni)

One woman whose natal family did not know her diagnosis, and another woman whose natal family was unaware of her husband's and her diagnoses, had not broached the topic of their children's future with them, since they felt that the natal families would wonder why they were making such a request and think it was out of the context, given the women's age. Both the women planned to reveal the diagnosis and solicit help for their children at a later date, though they had no doubt that their families would support them. The reason behind the postponement was that neither of them wanted to burden their natal families with the difficult news of HIV/AIDS until such time as they were severely ill and unable to manage on their own.

> Why should I tell my natal family (about the HIV diagnosis) now—they will only get upset to hear that we have this illness. Not that they will stay away—not that ... but they will feel very distressed that such a bad fate has fallen upon us, so why to unnecessarily trouble them? I have decided that as long as I can manage on my own, I will not tell them anything. Only when I am bed-ridden and cannot do for myself, then I will tell them. And now, without telling them about this AIDS, if I just ask them to see to the children in the future, they will wonder why I am making such a request

when I am young and healthy. So why create complications? I have said nothing to them so far—when the time is right, I will tell them about the illness and ask them to see to the children. They will support me, there is no doubt about that. (Diya)

Of these, one woman's children were adolescents and in her opinion needed guidance only, whereas the other woman's children were small and needed active rearing.

In addition, all the women were preoccupied with accumulating financial and/or material assets for their children. Also, four women whose husbands had property or who had property of their own were working towards/had already finished transferring this to their children. By providing their children with something of their own to fall back on, women felt that they were leaving no stone unturned in arranging for the well-being of their offspring after they passed away. To an extent, these efforts assuaged their distress about the uncertainty of their children's future.

Though I am looking after my health and trying to take care, side-by-side, I am planning for their (children's) future. Even though my (natal) family will see to them, I want them to have something of their own—somehow that makes me feel better, less uncertain about their future. So the house we have in the village—I have transferred it to the children's names ... that will come in useful for them at some time. (Falguni)

The women, however, did not mention anything about accumulating resources for their own future health needs.

Women had observed from close quarters what had happened to their husbands as the infection unfolded. They realised how much care their husbands had required at advanced stages, and they often wondered who would care for them the way they had done for their husbands. Even where they had shared their diagnosis with, and had assurances from, the natal family that the latter would look after them, women felt that given each one's own concerns and problems, as well as the demands of care in the HIV infection and of responsibility for their children, no one would care for them as they had for their husbands.

When he (husband) was ill, he needed so much of care, especially towards the end. And I did it all. Now I sometimes wonder who will care for me like that when I am ill? When he was ill, I was there so I did for him, but for me, who will do? My people (natal family) are there for me, but even so, how much can they do … work, look after their families, see to my daughter, see to me in an illness that just goes on getting worse? So this question comes to my mind. (Rima)

Learning Whom to Count on

Women's experiences with their social network and with the healthcare system, following the latter's knowledge of their husband's (and sometimes their own) diagnosis, made them realise whom they could turn to for support during the caregiving trajectory and as symptomatic positive women, formed another core theme.

For four women, the experience of learning whom they could count on started when their symptomatic husbands underwent the first HIV testing and were diagnosed seropositive, either in private nursing homes/clinics or in public-sector hospitals where they had been seeking treatment. Following the diagnosis, the refusal of these facilities to provide any further treatment and the transfer of the husband's case to a specific public-sector hospital (Hospital A), was the women's first realisation that they could not expect treatment everywhere.

One woman who was tested for HIV as a part of antenatal care (and when she was found to be positive, her husband was tested too), found that at Hospital J (a public hospital catering to the needs of expectant mothers) where she was seeking medical care during pregnancy, she continued to receive its services till the time of delivery. Following that she was told by some of the doctors at Hospital J that not every health centre looked after HIV/AIDS cases and hence, for follow-up treatment once symptoms started, she and her husband could go to NGO A with which the doctors were associated. According to the woman, the advice of the doctors made her realise that her options were limited in the case of this illness, as compared to other ones where she could exercise choice over the treatment centre. As a result of the doctor's advice, the woman and her husband never sought HIV-related treatment from the public-sector hospital (Hospital F) where the husband was employed.

Besides the transfer of treatment, doctors in the private health centres and staff of the public hospitals were found to share the seropositive diagnosis with relatives and/or acquaintances of the infected person, without the latter's knowledge or consent. As a result, it was inevitable that the news of the diagnosis would spread within the social network. For four women, it was the news of their husband's diagnosis that spread, while for the woman receiving antenatal care, it was the news of both her and her husband's diagnoses.

Among the first four women, for one, such violations of confidentiality guidelines by the staff in Hospital K (a public hospital) were responsible for her in-laws, who resided in Mumbai, getting to know of her husband's seropositive status. Indeed, when a member of this woman's natal family (who were based in the native village in North India) came to stay with her and her children and help them out on being informed that the husband was ill and in hospital, similar disclosure practices resulted in him hearing the husband's seropositive diagnosis and informing the rest of the natal household.

In a second case, the woman's neighbourhood got to know of the husband's seropositive diagnosis almost immediately, once again due to the disregard of confidentiality principles in a private hospital. In this instance, the in-law and natal families, who lived in the native village in North India, were informed of the husband's seropositivity by the woman herself, when she and her family relocated there in order to get family support for her caregiving role and to transfer her husband's property to her children.

A third woman's in-laws who resided in Mumbai became aware of her husband's serostatus, but not the natal family who were in the native village, some hours from Mumbai. In this woman's case, her husband, prior to showing his test result to the doctor, showed it to his employer. In the absence of pre-test and post-test counselling, he had no idea of the implications of his action. His employer, on seeing the report, not only terminated his services in an indirect manner by repeatedly and insistently asking him to go on leave, but also shared the diagnosis with other employees. It was only when the HIV-positive person met his doctor (a private medical practitioner) that he understood what had happened, but here too the doctor shared the diagnosis with the positive person in the presence of the latter's brother, and hence his family of origin also got to know of his positive status. This person, as indicated earlier, started serving liquor in his home in order to earn a living.

In the fourth case, both the in-laws and natal family, based in Mumbai, besides the entire workplace and neighbourhood, heard about the husband's serostatus. Here, the husband worked as a permanent employee in a public hospital (Hospital H) and lived in quarters on the hospital premises. Doctors at the private nursing home where the husband had been tested informed a workplace acquaintance of the positive person about the test result. Not only did this person spread the news among the infected person's natal and in-law families, but also among his employers, colleagues and neighbours. While the continuity of the positive person's employment was not affected since his department head was very understanding and knew that given the nature of his job, his presence did not endanger anybody, discrimination from all (except one) co-workers and their families, resulting in a sense of isolation at work and at home, as well as a refusal to provide treatment in Hospital H, were reported.

In the case of the woman whose testing was done during antenatal care, her natal and in-law families who lived in Mumbai were informed of both her and her husband's positive status by the staff of Hospital J, a public hospital where she was seeking antenatal care.

For two women, then, the news of HIV-seropositivity was confined to their relatives, but for three women, this was not so.

Since the four women whose husbands were tested before them transferred the latter's treatment to Hospital A, they underwent testing there. Hospital A was known for maintaining ethical standards and a supportive attitude towards positive people, and hence the confidentiality of the women's seropositivity was maintained. Yet, since the in-laws of three women knew the husbands' diagnosis, they asked whether the wife was positive. Besides, two of these women informed their natal families of their serostatus but one did not. A fourth woman who relocated to her native village in North India during the caregiving trajectory was asked by the doctor treating her husband there whether she too was positive, and on getting an affirmative reply, informed her in-laws. However, the natal family remained unaware of her seropositive state.

Thus for three women, the in-laws and the natal family knew both the husband's and the wife's diagnoses; for one, the in-laws were aware of both the husband's and the wife's diagnoses whereas the natal family had heard of the husband's; and for the fifth woman, the in-laws knew both spouses' diagnoses but the natal family had no idea of either. The news of the husbands' diagnosis had spread among the neighbourhood for one couple; among the workplace for one; and among the workplace and neighbourhood, which were located on the same premises, for one (see Table 6.2).

As stated above, four women whose husbands were already symptomatic at the time of testing took their husbands to Hospital A for treatment. Since Hospital A was located at one end of the city, having to obtain treatment from there was perceived as difficult because of the indirect costs involved, and the physical strain that travelling such a distance put on the positive person. Moreover, when husbands were severely ill and unable to travel such long distances in public transport, women had to arrange for transport through private taxis, hiking up the indirect costs many times over.

> After the doctors in ____ (a private nursing home where testing was done) told us to go to Hospital A, I began to take him (husband) there. But it was very tough because Hospital A is so far, at the other end of the city. As it were, taking public transport in Mumbai is very expensive, and on top of that, he was so weak that it was hard for him to travel so much, that too in the crowded buses and trains. When he could not move much, then I used to take him by taxi and that would cost Rs 250 or so, one way, so you can imagine .... It was really very, very difficult ... such limited treatment facilities, that too in one corner of the city. (Rima)

Though the staff of Hospital A was seen as supportive in its attitude, and, understanding the limited resources the women had, put all of them in touch with NGO D for assistance, the facilities at Hospital A itself were not rated very highly. Though it

Table 6.2

Locating the spread of the seropositive diagnoses of caregiving wives and their husbands

Participant	Spread of husband's diagnosis to in-laws	Spread of own diagnosis to in-laws	Spread of husband's diagnosis to natal family	Spread of own diagnosis to natal family	Spread of husband's diagnosis to workplace/ neighbourhood	Spread of own diagnosis to workplace/ neighbourhood
1	Yes	Yes	Yes	Yes	Workplace and neighbourhood	No
2	Yes	Yes	No	No	Workplace	No
3	Yes	Yes	Yes	Yes	No	No
4	Yes	Yes	Yes	No	Neighbourhood	No
5	Yes	Yes	Yes	Yes	No	No

was a public hospital which provided free service and was known for its HIV-related services, quite often only consultation would be free since medicines were sometimes not available in the dispensary and diagnostic facilities were at times in a dysfunctional condition. Medicines and diagnostic tests then had to be sought from other sources, which NGO D helped out with through networking with relevant organisations from whom free/concessional services were obtained.

> You know how these government hospitals are ... so Hospital A was like that. Of course, the good thing was that the doctors and nurses, other staff were very nice, they never kept you away because you had this AIDS and so on. In fact, they were always very understanding, very comforting ... they only put us in touch with these NGO D people because they could see our circumstances. But sometimes the medicines were not there, the X-ray machine would be broken ... so treatment would become a problem. But once NGO D people were helping us, then they would make alternative arrangements. (Falguni)

Due to the high indirect costs, one family stopped seeking treatment for the husband from Hospital A, preferring to rely on their family doctor, even though this meant that they had to bear the direct costs themselves, since NGO D's intervention did not reimburse private healthcare intervention. The doctor who had initially transferred the case to Hospital A later agreed to provide treatment, and his support and cooperation were considered to be excellent. Not only did he give good treatment, but he also provided emotional courage.

> Initially after he (husband) was diagnosed with AIDS, we went to Hospital A for treatment. But it was so expensive going all the way there, the entire day would be spent in travelling and waiting, and the cost was so high even by public transport, that ____ (husband) said that he would rather go to ____ (our family doctor) here itself. The doctor had initially told us to go to Hospital A for treatment, but when we explained to him how difficult it was for us to go over there, he agreed to help us out. So till the end, we went

to him only. He was very good to us ... used to give us a lot of courage, tell us not to give up, to look after ourselves. He would examine him, give injections with disposable needles ... so he had no problems as such. Of course, we had to pay him ourselves, the NGO D people said that they did not give money for private treatment. But we felt it was all right since we did not have the strain of travelling so much and wasting the whole day—and the travel money went to the doctor, you could say. (Diya)

One woman who moved to her native village in North India for family support and property-related matters in the later stages of her husband's illness, used the services of a private medical doctor there. The doctor provided treatment despite knowing the diagnosis, but refused to examine the patient or to touch him. Nonetheless, the woman considered herself to be lucky. In her view, doctors in rural areas, being unaware of diseases such as HIV/AIDS, harbour many misconceptions because of which they refuse to treat such patients. That she was able to locate a doctor who understood the infection better than other doctors in the village, and who was willing to help her out, was such a relief that his refusal to touch and examine the seropositive person did not become a major issue.

You know how it is in the villages ... doctors are backward, they do not know much, not like the Mumbai doctors. They have false ideas about so many illnesses. So when the doctor agreed to treat my husband even though he read on the case paper that he had AIDS, it was such a relief. He made it clear from the beginning that he would not examine him or touch him but I felt that it was OK because at least, he agreed to treat him—and that way, he was very helpful and understanding. (Sona)

Husbands in two cases required hospitalisation in the post-diagnosis period, one of them repeatedly. While one husband was hospitalised in Hospital A, the other initially was admitted to Hospital H, a public-sector hospital where he worked and lived, but because of discriminatory practices there, he turned to Hospital A.

The fifth woman and her husband were asymptomatic at the time of testing. Symptoms began in the husband about a year later and, as instructed by doctors at Hospital J, the wife took him to NGO A for treatment. NGO A was an out-patient intervention facility, providing free medical consultation and some assistance with diagnostic tests and treatment, either through providing these services free or networking with other centres to provide these services at concessional rates/as free. NGO A was known as a place where HIV-positive people were treated with support, and emotional care was an important component of intervention. For the woman accessing its services, NGO A was located near her in-law's residence where she resided during the husband's life-time, and hence indirect costs at that time were minimal. Over-all, she reported satisfaction with her experiences at NGO A.

> When he (husband) started falling ill, then as per the doc-tors' instruction at the time of my pregnancy, I took him to NGO A. It is located very near my in-law's house, where we were staying at that time, so going there was not a problem for us. They used to give all their services free and they were very nice people—they would help us out with our problems, give a lot of courage ... if we had to have some treatment or test that they could not provide, then they would ask some other centre to give this either at less cost or free, so in that way, they would help us a lot. (Urvashi)

For the purpose of hospitalisation, NGO A staff recommended this woman's husband to public hospitals G and I, but due to discrim-inatory practices at the former, the family relied on Hospital I.

Hospitalisation in Hospitals A and I was without event, since patients and their families were dealt with without discrimina-tion. However, as discussed earlier, for wives it did not mean a break in caregiving since the staff provided limited assistance and families were still expected to see to the patients. Caregivers, therefore, found that instead of providing them with respite from caregiving, hospitalisation added to their strain.

During hospitalisation in Hospitals H and G, husbands experi-enced discrimination. For instance, one husband who was seek-ing out-patient care from Hospital A decided to get in-patient care from Hospital H, where he worked and lived. He believed that being hospitalised in Hospital H would enable his wife to combine her household, child care and caregiving roles more easily, since the hospital and the home were located on the same premises. However, since the news of his diagnosis had spread throughout the workplace and neighbourhood, the staff of the ward where he was admitted knew about it and informed the other inmates who protested against his presence, requesting the doctor on duty to discharge him. Though the doctor on duty left the decision to his superior, the latter did discharge him but explained to the couple that treating him at Hospital H, was not possible and that they should go to Hospital A, where specialists in HIV/AIDS practised. The seropositive individual and his wife were deeply disturbed by the experience.

> Sometime after he (husband) was diagnosed and we were taking treatment from Hospital A, he began to get some swelling because of a TB lump. The Hospital A doctors wanted him to get admitted to get it aspirated. But he decided to have it done here in Hospital H because he felt that since we live right here, it will be helpful for me to see to him, the child and the house. But when he was admitted here, since the news of his diagnosis had spread everywhere in Hospital H, the nurse in the ward knew about it and she told all the other patients about it in the night. They called the RMO (resident medical officer) who was on duty and asked that he be removed. But the RMO would not do anything till he consulted the main doctor. When the main doctor came in the morning, he discharged him saying that we should go to Hospital A for treatment because there were specialists there and Hospital H could not help out for this disease. We felt very bad about it, very, very sad. Why should they do like that? (Rima)

Women reported that they were upset with the refusals they encountered from healthcare centres, as well as with the violations of confidentiality and discrimination during hospitalisation. They believed that the healthcare system was meant to help them and not create further problems for them. However, they did nothing about it, not only because they were too caught up with trying to manage a difficult situation and to survive, but also because they had no idea of where to turn to for redressal.

One goes to a hospital or a doctor with such hope ... one expects to be cured and to be helped. But here, instead of that, you get not only a death statement but they ruin your whole life by refusing to help, by telling others and causing all sorts of problems. We were so upset ... none of our neighbours would talk to us, we had to go all the way to Hospital A for treatment ... but what to do? There was no choice and we had to manage somehow. Whom can we tell these things to? Even if there is someone, who had the time then? So we just plodded on with our problems and with our pain. (Sona)

As mentioned earlier, four women were receiving support from NGO D. Through its programme to support children living in HIV-affected homes, NGO D provided families belonging to particular income groups with nutritional support, support for the education of children, medical support, networking with medical centres, emotional support though group meetings and individual counselling, home visits and visits during hospitalisation, as well as legal services relating to child custody. Women could also contact the NGO staff telephonically during times of need/crises and they would respond appropriately.

Since the women had to arrange for resources on their own for the care of their husbands and for the survival of their families, when severe illness episodes in the husbands hampered the latter's ability to earn and caregiving demands and household responsibilities prevented women from taking up paid employment outside the home, the medical, nutritional and educational support of NGO D was seen as an important contribution to family survival during the lifetime of the husband, when HIV/AIDS had unleashed economic hardship on the family.

When he (husband) was very ill, I could not work. And afterwards, his salary was also cut because he did not have leave. At that time we had so many financial problems and I had to borrow money ... so when we started getting help from NGO D, it was really a blessing for us, otherwise, managing was very hard. Their support helped us a lot, or how would we have survived? Milk, medicines, ration money, food items, money for ___ (child's) education—all that they gave us. If the medicines or tests could not be done at Hospital A, they would put us in touch with doctors they knew for free treatment .... So they did a lot. And their help eased my burden. Of course, it did not take care of everything, because they give help for specific things, and other things, one has to manage. But still, it made a lot of difference. Because of this, our need to borrow was reduced. Plus, you feel that someone is there for you. (Rima)

Women were happy not just with the medical, material and financial services, but also with the emotional care that they received from the staff. Staff not only lent a patient ear to the women's problems, but also explored various solutions and alternatives, implementing the most appropriate one. Reassuring the women about their continued presence made the latter feel a sense of connectedness. Providing hope about, and courage to face, the future were also important components of emotional care.

NGO D people's help ... how can one describe it? One knew that they would be there and it was so reassuring ... like they would visit us often at home, spend time with us to understand how we were, what we needed ... if anything happened, we just had to phone them and they would come. Or if we went there for meetings or to collect the rations or reimbursements, they would spend time with us individually and listen to us. When he (husband) was in the hospital, they would come there too, with fruits ... spend time with us. They would always give us a lot of courage, hope ... help us to plan the future. So you felt that someone was there, someone cared. (Rima)

Interactions with other women in similar positions at NGO D's group meetings not only helped the women realise that there were others facing experiences like theirs, but they also learnt from them. From the stories of other women, the participants not only got a glimpse into the illness and caregiving trajectories, but also learnt about various ways of dealing with difficult situations and about the reliability of NGO D staff in being there for them.

They (NGO D) used to have these group meetings. When he (husband) was not so ill, I would go for the group meetings—

there I could meet other women, and share my experiences, and learn from theirs ... what happens, how to manage, how NGO D people would help out ... we would all give each other courage. I used to feel better to know that there were others like me, it made me feel less alone. And the staff would be there and advise us. I learnt a lot and got a lot of comfort from these meetings. (Rima)

Three women reported receiving a lot of assistance, especially emotional support, from the staff of NGO D around the time of, and immediately before and after, the deaths of their husbands.

From the women's narratives, it was clear that though the services of NGO D were not designed with the caregiving role in mind, they facilitated role performance in various ways. Medical and network support helped in the provision of clinical treatment, while nutritional support allowed for the maintenance of health status. Individual and group counselling eased caregiver distress, helped find solutions to various problems and prepared caregivers for what lay ahead of them—in other words, caregiver coping was enhanced. Nutritional and educational support also helped the women in looking after their family's needs.

Following the deaths of their husbands, the four women continued to receive the same support from NGO D as they had been doing earlier. Though the women were now earning for their families, nutritional and educational support from NGO D was still valued since it supplemented their incomes. Medical support was reassured, though the women required this only later, since in the initial post-death phase they remained asymptomatic. Besides this, they were helped to adjust to their position as widows and single parents, and encouraged to take a greater interest in the maintenance of their own health. Women reported discussing their plans for the future of their children with the NGO staff, who were seen as helping them weigh out and decide on alternatives. Women described themselves as feeling reassured that the NGO D staff would continue to provide material and educational support for their children even after they had passed away. Emotional support continued to form a significant component of NGO D's intervention.

With symptom onset, two women sought treatment from Hospital A. The woman who moved in with her natal family was now located far away from NGO A, but she still followed up with them since she often visited her shop which was located near NGO A. She also went on a payment basis to a private doctor located near her natal family for treatment, but he was not informed of her serostatus for fear that he would stop treatment and inform others of her infection.

> When I fall ill, then I go to this doctor here ... in private ... because it is nearby ... NGO A is far away from here and it is not always convenient for me to go there. But I have not told him about this AIDS. Why to unnecessarily cause trouble for myself and my family? I only tell him that it is fever, diarrhoea, like that. But once in 3–4 weeks, I anyway visit NGO A because I go to my shop and NGO A is just five minutes from there, so they know how my condition is, they monitor my progress. (Urvashi)

A fourth woman who got a permanent job in the public hospital where her husband had been working (Hospital H) sought treatment from there itself. This woman was aware that she was taking a risk by doing so since the news of her husband's diagnosis (but not hers) had spread throughout the hospital premises, which resulted in both the hospital authorities and staff knowing about it; hence, there was a possibility that they suspected her of being infected too, though this had not been an issue at the time of her appointment, when neither employers nor co-workers had asked her serostatus nor recommended her for testing. Yet, she believed that seeking treatment from Hospital A was too cumbersome to manage, not only because it was too far away and would require her to take leave from work to do so, but because it would also interrupt her routine of accompanying her daughter to and from school. She therefore preferred to seek treatment from Hospital H itself, and while she never revealed her serostatus to healthcare personnel there, she was always prepared for the possibility that they may ask her about it or recommend/insist that she do an HIV test. She was quite clear that not only would she lie about her serostatus if questioned about it, but also that she would revert to Hospital A for treatment if she was asked to get herself tested.

When I get fever, diarrhoea, I go to Hospital H itself. Hospital A is so far ... means I have to take leave, then what about her (child's) school and so on? So this is very convenient. Of course, the fear is there because everyone knew that my husband had AIDS, so I always have the worry that they may ask me to get tested ... that way no one had referred to my health when I had applied for the job or when I got it, even now no one says anything ... but you never know when the topic may come up, since they knew about him ... so that fear is always there but if they ask me, I will not tell them and I will not do the test, I will go to Hospital A for treatment. (Rima)

According to the women, withdrawal was the uniform response from their in-laws when the latter heard the seropositive diagnoses.

His (husband's) people just stopped bothering about us once they got to know he had AIDS. They live just nearby and could see me struggling to look after him and the children, and to manage the house and earn, but they never once inquired. I needed some help sometimes but what to do? (Diya)

In the case of the woman who had been pregnant at the time of testing, since she was tested before her husband, the in-law family believed that she was responsible for contracting the infection and giving it to their son. Thus, though the infected couple and their first child continued to live with the in-laws till the time of the husband's death, they experienced hostility and lack of support.

When they (the in-laws) heard that we had this illness, they at once blamed me for it because I had been tested first. They began to behave very badly with us, not speaking, not letting us touch things in the house ... when he fell ill, they never helped me look after him, even though we were living with them. They knew that I was also having the same problem and had to take care of myself but they never helped me. Their idea was that I was responsible for the infection and I was responsible for his care. The only thing was that they did not ask us to leave the house. (Urvashi)

For the other three women whose in-laws initially heard of the husband's diagnosis and later the wife's, they minimised their contact with the family. They rarely visited them and offered no support at all, though wives kept them informed when the husband's condition deteriorated. Wives believed that it was their duty to keep the in-laws posted so that they could not be held responsible later for not having done so.

> When his (husband's) family got to know that we had this illness, they hardly bothered about us ... they would come over very rarely and not show any concern, they never asked if we needed anything ... but whatever it is, I would always keep them informed about his health, his progress—I would phone them or I would send a message. Finally they should not say that I had not told them ... after all, he is their son, so if I don't tell them, they will say that it was because of me that they did not know. So I always informed them. It made no difference to their attitude, but at least, I was doing my duty. (Rima)

The fifth woman whose in-law and natal families both lived in the native village in North India, decided to return there when her husband grew very ill. Since the news of her husband's diagnosis had spread in the neighbourhood, which had led to the complete withdrawal of all acquaintances and friends, she had to manage on her own in the city and so, the woman believed that if she returned to the village, the in-laws and natal family would help her and she could also ensure the transfer of her husband's property to her children. However, on hearing the husband's diagnosis, the in-laws withdrew all support except for reluctantly allowing her to stay in the family house. They also refused to transfer the property, saying that they would do so when the children became adults, causing doubts in the woman's mind as to whether this would really happen or not.

> Here (in Mumbai) when we got to know that he (husband) had this AIDS, the whole neighbourhood also got to know and no one was willing to have anything to do with us. When he grew seriously ill also, I was completely on my own. I decided then that it was better for us to go to the village, because at least both our families were there, they would help us. I also wanted to make the property in the children's

name when he was alive because it is easier if he dealt with his brothers—he was getting worse and I felt that the children would have some security if the property was transferred. So we went to the village. But when we told them that he had AIDS, they became very nasty with us—they would say do not touch this, do not let him use the bathroom ... they would not help me look after him, it was my brothers who helped. And they wanted us to return to Mumbai, not to stay in their house. But I told them that since he had a right to stay there, we would not budge—so they reluctantly agreed. But they would not transfer the property, they went on saying that only once the children turned 21 ... we fought so much with them but they would not listen ... even now, it has not been transferred and I am very worried about this...what will happen? (Sona)

During the lifetime of their husbands, then, women received no support from their in-laws for their caregiving role and family related responsibilities, nor were they assisted in maintaining their own health status, though the in-laws knew that they were positive. This attitude continued even at the time of the husband's death, where in-laws showed reluctance to meet the husband and spend time with him when informed that the end was near, even if they were staying in the same house. Further, in-laws showed little interest in assisting with and paying for funeral rites, and it was the wife's natal family who took up the responsibility.

The in-laws remained like this till the end—they just did not bother. Everything was left to me, though they knew that I was having AIDS also and the doctors at Hospital J had told them that I also needed to take care of my health. They could see me running around but they just insisted that I was the wife, it was my job. Even at the end, when he (husband) was in Hospital I and I phoned them to come as doctors had given up hope, they took so long to come. They just did not care. (Urvashi)

Following the death of the husbands, the in-laws continued to behave in the same manner with the wives and their children. Besides the minimal contact and complete lack of support, disputes over property were reported by two women. In the first case, the woman stated that her in-law family refused to transfer the husband's share of the property to her children and at the time of data collection, the wife was still struggling to get it, while in another, the in-law family attempted to take back the husband's property (which was already in his name) from the wife and her refusal to give it back led to the in-laws making her and her child leave the house.

> After he (husband) died, then they (in-laws) began to ask me for the shop back—this was in his name and they wanted it. But I refused—it was all I had to manage with in the future. So they fought very badly with me but I flatly refused, and so they told me to get out of the house. (Urvashi)

Even after the death of their sons, the in-law families refused to recognise the vulnerability of their daughters-in-law and to respond with compassion towards them.

The behaviour of the in-laws troubled the women. While they were not completely surprised at the in-laws' attitude towards themselves, given the deep-seated cultural orientation that daughters-in-law are outsiders and so cannot be trusted, they could not understand how the in-laws could abandon their sons who were their own flesh and blood. Moreover, women were bewildered as to how the in-laws could maintain such a hostile stand during a crisis when support was of utmost importance. The women were sure that the in-laws had understood the gravity of the situation and yet chose to distance themselves.

> And those people (in-laws), even after knowing that he (husband) was so ill, didn't ask a single word. Once they knew he had this illness, they hardly came and never, ever bothered. Their own son ... but they did not care at all. Everything was left to me. Naturally, one will feel it. When one has parents and they do not bother to even inquire about their own child, won't one feel? I just cannot understand it .... With me, of course, they would not bother because that is how women are seen, daughters-in-law have no standing ... but how can one reject one's own child to such an extent? That too, at such times, when death is around the corner. (Rima)

At the same time, the women realised that the negative perceptions of the infection, the fear that they (the in-laws) would have to undertake the expenditure for a long and incapacitating illness (though most of them could afford it), fear that they would have to look after the son's family during his incapacitation and after his death and share the family property with them, as well as fear that they would have to look after the seropositive wife when she became symptomatic, motivated the in-laws' behaviour. Wives also got the impression that the in-laws held them responsible for getting the infection and passing it on to the son. According to the wives, the in-laws felt that since they (the wives) were the cause of the problem, they should also be the ones to take the consequences.

> They (in-laws) were worried that they would have to do everything for us—look after him (husband), pay for his treatment, see to me and my daughter. Then later they would have to look after me and my daughter, and I was also infected, so I would soon be as sick as my husband and then, after my death, they would have to do everything for my daughter. The other thing was property ... because they did not want to give me my share of the property ... so that was why they became so indifferent. That too they knew very well that he had infected me with his loose ways but my mother-in-law insisted that I had done something at my mother's place and come—she never considered her son to be at fault. So obviously, she would not want to help me out. The attitude was that since I got the infection into the house, I should see to the problems. (Urvashi)

Anger in the two women whose in-laws attempted/were attempting to deprive them and their children of their share of the property was clearly evident. These women were aware that the property was rightfully theirs and/or their children's, and it disturbed them greatly to realise that their in-laws were trying to usurp it from them. The woman whose property transfer was still to be settled was determined to ensure that the process was completed as soon as possible, because she feared that if she passed away without doing so, her children would lose their claim.

I want to go to the village and put the property in the children's names. These people (in-laws) are saying that they will do it when the children become 21, but who can wait till then? If I die before that, then they will not give it to the children. So I want to make sure about it. The children have a right because it is their father's, but these people are trying to act smart and rob them of it. I am very anxious about this because it has to be done soon—I really worry and worry about it because if the children lose it then they will have nothing to fall back on. These children have already lost their father and now these people want to take the property also—what to say? I feel so cheated. (Sona)

Natal families of the women who knew the diagnoses of both the spouses or of the husband responded supportively, providing whatever support they could, depending on their own capacity and on the needs of the women and their families. Knowing that the women were innocent victims who were in no way responsible for acquiring the infection, natal families rallied around them.

My (natal) family knows that I am innocent in all this. They know what I am like, and that I have done nothing to get this disease. They know that my husband is responsible. They know how much I have suffered and how my in-laws have treated me. That is why they have shown me so much concern, that is why when I came back to my mother's house after his death, they welcomed me with open arms. (Urvashi)

During the lifetime of the husbands, two women reported receiving emotional, material and financial support spontaneously from their natal families who knew their predicament and understood their needs. Further, one woman, who as mentioned earlier had returned to the native village in North India with her ill husband and children, received emotional support and assistance with caregiving from her natal family who was too poor to provide material/financial help. Additionally, in these three cases, the natal families assisted with caregiving through accompanying the couple to the doctor, and if required, looking after children when the husband was in hospital and the wife was seeing to him there.

Members of the natal family would stay with the wives when the end was near, and took charge of funeral arrangements as well.

> My brothers stood by me. They helped me to look after him (husband). They came with me to the doctor, ran around for things I needed. They were very understanding and boosted my spirits all the time. Though they are too poor to help me with money, they were there for me in every other way. They knew how hard my life had been and so when I told them what had happened, they immediately came to my aid. When he died, they were present and they saw to all the arrangements. The in-laws did not even want to enter the room—even after informing that he was nearing the end, they did not bother to visit till the last minute. (Sona)

For a fourth woman whose natal family lived in the native village in North India, a male member of the family came to Mumbai to assist her when she informed them that her husband was very ill and in hospital. At the time of informing the natal family, the husband was admitted at Hospital K, a public hospital, and he had not yet been tested for HIV. By the time the natal family member arrived in Mumbai, the husband had been tested and found to be positive, and was to be transferred to Hospital A for further treatment. It was from the staff of Hospital K that the natal family member got to know the husband's seropositive diagnosis and informed the natal family about it. Soon after, on getting her own test result, the woman informed her natal family of her own seropositivity. Nonetheless, the natal family continued to support the woman, her husband and her children. Not only did they send considerable money, but their representative also stayed with the woman's family in Mumbai, looking after her children while she cared for her husband in the hospital (which in the post-diagnosis period, was Hospital A). The man also worked in Mumbai while assisting the family, and his income was used for their needs. When the husband passed away three months later, he returned to the village.

The support of the natal families continued after the death of the husbands. After being made to leave her in-law's home over a property dispute, one woman was welcomed back to the natal home. She enjoyed the support of her natal family though she was economically independent. The natal families of the other three women also opened their doors to them, though for various reasons discussed earlier, the women chose to retain independent units. Since these women began earning and continued to receive help from the NGO D, they refused to accept material and financial help from their natal families, as highlighted previously. Seeing that the women were able to manage with their incomes and with NGO D's help, natal families acceded to their wishes. However, emotional reassurance that they cared about them and could be counted on at all times was constantly given. Moreover, where natal families knew the women's diagnosis, they willingly agreed to care for their children in the future, repeatedly reassuring the women and directing them not to worry on this count.

As described in the previous theme, when symptoms set in, the woman living with her natal family received care from them. One woman, whose natal family lived in the neighbouring suburb, decided to manage on her own as she felt that she had troubled the natal family enough. Moreover, her symptoms were very mild and so self-management was possible. There were two women whose natal families were both in native villages in North India, and hence it was difficult for them to help out during symptomatic periods. While one of these women whose illness episodes were accompanied by considerable weakness and hence required some care, was looked after by her adolescent sons, the other woman managed on her own. Here too, self-care was possible since symptoms were mild.

Women deeply appreciated the support of their natal families. Having experienced rejection from the in-law family and indifference from their husbands, and given the cultural attitude that married daughters no longer belong to the natal home, and in some cases knowing the economic position and other problems of the family of origin, women realised the value of the natal family's support. They knew that if their natal families had not come to their rescue, they would have no one to care for them.

> If it were not for my people (natal family), I do not know where I would be. You know, no one was bothered about me and my family when we got this AIDS problem—but my people were there. They have their own problems but they never let that come in the way. In fact, they are so far away

but my brother-in-law especially came ... he stayed here, worked here just to help me out ... they sent me money—even now, they show so much concern, tell me to look after myself, tell me not to worry about the children. Because I know that they are there for me, I can go on. What they do means a lot to me because you know in our culture how a married daughter is seen. I can never thank them enough. (Falguni)

One woman did not disclose her and her husband's diagnoses to her natal family, who lived in the native village located four to five hours from Mumbai. Her opinion was that though she knew her natal family would continue to support her despite the knowledge of the diagnoses, she did not wish to burden them with such difficult news for as long as she could manage independently. She therefore maintained it as a secret. When the husband grew ill, she told her natal family that he had TB, and they helped her out with financial assistance and emotional support during the illness and caregiving trajectories. Due to the geographical distance, support with caregiving tasks was possible only during the periods when the natal family visited.

At the time when the husband was totally incapacitated, he expressed a desire to go to the woman's natal family in the village, though the wife was unclear as to the exact reason behind the request. Nonetheless, honouring his wishes, the wife arranged for this. The husband passed away at the wife's natal home a day after reaching there. The natal family extended all support and care during the day he was alive, and also took care of funeral arrangements and expenses. The in-law family, located in Mumbai, had not only minimised contact with the positive person and his family, following the knowledge of the seropositive diagnoses, but had also shown a reluctance to visit them when they were in their home in Mumbai and had been informed by the wife that the husband was completely debilitated. On being informed of the death of the husband, the in-laws delayed going to the woman's natal village for the last rites, and did not offer to undertake funeral-related expenses and arrangements.

Even in the post-death phase, the woman did not reveal her diagnosis to her natal family, maintaining that she did not wish to trouble them till it became unavoidable. Thus, though her natal family welcomed her back into their home after the passing away of her husband, she preferred to return to the city where her children were studying and where she could get good treatment when she became symptomatic. She returned to the city and lived independently with her children, managing to earn by continuing her husband's alcohol business. She remained asymptomatic till the time of data collection, and decided to defer the disclosure of seropositivity and request for support for the future of her children for as long as she could manage. Contact between her and the natal family remained close and affectionate, with emotional support and occasional visits from their side.

When the news of a husband's diagnosis spread to the neighbourhood, it resulted in one family experiencing complete hostility from those around them. As stated earlier, while this prompted the wife's decision to relocate to the native village in North India during her husband's severe symptomatic phase so that she could receive support from her in-law and natal families who lived there, on her return to Mumbai after the death of her husband, she settled in another part of the city where her family's past history and health status were not known.

Another woman, whose husband's diagnosis had spread to both the workplace and the neighbourhood located on the same premises of Hospital H, reported that during her husband's lifetime, her family experienced discrimination from all except one family who was sympathetic and continued to interact with her. Besides showing concern and giving courage, this family responded to her occasional requests to help arrange transport for visits to Hospital A when the husband was very ill and could not use public transport, as well as to line up people to carry the husband down the stairs when he was too ill to walk. At the time of the husband's death, this family kept the couple's young daughter in their home, so that she could be spared the trauma of watching her father die. In the post-death phase, while this family remained solicitous of the wife and child, offering to help whenever required, others in the neighbourhood and workplace (which became the woman's workplace after she began working at the hospital), were no longer hostile. Whereas no one knew the wife's diagnosis, hospital authorities did not raise it as an issue for her appointment, nor did employees and neighbours bring it up as a possibility.

A woman, whose husband's and whose own diagnoses were known to the in-law family and whose husband's diagnosis was known to people at the husband's former workplace, described receiving spontaneous support from her neighbours as well as occasional financial assistance from her husband's former boss. No experiences of discrimination from his former colleagues were reported. During her husband's lifetime, seeing the woman struggle to manage the multiple roles of caregiving, child rearing and earning single-handedly, neighbours would inquire about what was wrong with the husband and offer to help her with her tasks. Comfort and hope during the worsening of the husband's condition were also given. While the woman never divulged the diagnosis to her neighbours, but claimed that her husband was suffering from TB, she appreciated their concern. Since she had to manage so many roles at once, she sometimes requested neighbours to keep an eye on her husband during bouts of severe illness when she went to drop and fetch her children from school, or to make any purchases. Following the death of her husband, neighbours always assured her of their presence and protection, making her feel less insecure about living alone with her children. The former employer of the woman's husband had terminated the latter's services on knowing his serostatus. However, he visited the family occasionally, giving them money when he did so. This continued till the positive person was alive. On hearing of his passing away, the employer visited the bereaved family, once again giving them some money. He also told the wife that she could approach him for money whenever she required, though he did not visit the family after that.

While women learnt whom they could count on, they also reported a sense of discomfort with their dependence. They believed that at their age, they should be independent and should not have to trouble others with their problems. While the length of time over which they required support added to their discomfort, sociocultural norms indicating that married women no longer belong to the natal family, and should manage on their own in their marital homes without relying on their families of origin, made them feel even more awkward. However, women realised that support was indispensable under the circumstances, and were deeply grateful to have received it and benefited from it, indicating how important it was for their future and that of their children.

Many times, I feel very ashamed because I need help from others. I always feel that at my age, I should be independent,

I should manage on my own. Life has no meaning if one goes on taking from others. But what to do? If I had not taken from NGO D and from my people (natal family), we would have not survived, my daughter would have no future. So I have no choice really. But it embarrasses me ... you know how it is in our culture—girls should be on their own once they are married. (Rima)

That women reported feelings of aloneness throughout their interface with HIV/AIDS, despite the support they were receiving, was an important finding that was difficult to explain. Women themselves were unable to explain their paradoxical experience. One woman hypothesised that perhaps it was because ultimately they had to live out the experience themselves and support could not obliterate the pain and difficulties involved, suggesting that everyone has private spaces that others cannot enter even if they try, and that one cannot always escape from these even if one wishes to do so.

I feel very alone. Even though my (natal) family is there and has stood by me throughout, NGO D is with me and has done so much for me, I still feel alone. After all, it is one's own life, one's own experience, which no one else can live— I have to go through it on my own. (Rima)

Finally, women reported that as a result of managing the challenges posed by HIV/AIDS, they realised how strong and resilient they were. Prior to this, they had not been aware of the extent of their capabilities. Moreover, having been able to manage under such difficult circumstances made women look at themselves with greater respect and admiration.

I myself am so surprised that I have been able to manage such a tough situation, that too almost single-handedly. I had no idea that I could do so much, that I could be so strong. I look at myself and think that earlier I had never felt that I could handle such challenges, but now that I have, I know my true capabilities. And it is a good feeling I have about myself. (Falguni)

7 | THE WAY FORWARD

Across the globe, family care is a topic of immense contemporary significance because of a growing number of families who provide care to chronically ill, disabled and elderly members. The deinstitutionalisation movement, policies of community care and progress in medical science have all contributed to this emerging phenomenon (Seltzer and Heller 1997). Influenced by international developments, family care is being promoted in India too. India's adoption of the structural adjustment programme (SAP) has resulted in cutbacks in health sector expenditure and adoption of policies of community care. This transfers the responsibility of care for ill people to their families, adversely affecting the micro-environment of the household (Qadeer 2000) and unleashing severe financial strain, especially for poor families (Prabhu 2000). Such an approach is implemented in the context of HIV/AIDS as well, despite the infection's pandemic proportions in the country, its unique demands stemming from its complex psychosocial character, and its devastating impact on families.

Studies of the family experience of HIV/AIDS (for example, Bharat 1996 and D'Cruz 2003a) show that families looking after seropositive members experience altered dynamics, economic setbacks, deteriorating quality of life as well as caregiving burden. This book has highlighted the dynamics of family care in HIV/AIDS and contributes to our knowledge in several ways. Incorporating van Manen's hermeneutic phenomenological approach, the book has captured the lived experience of ten caregivers (including five seropositive caregivers) and seven care receivers in Mumbai, India. Countering the criticisms of family care research and of studies examining family care in HIV/AIDS, the present work has covered aspects such as care receiving, emotional support and the organisation of care within families, in relation to a range of family forms and life-cycle stages, as well as, economic classes. The adoption of a phenomenological approach is also relevant in this regard since it helps us grasp the essence of a phenomenon and makes explicit the structure of meaning of the experience.

Findings of the study indicate that the essential structure of care receiver experiences was captured in two key themes, namely, losing autonomy and redefining family relationships. The core of seronegative caregivers' experiences centred around their struggle to prolong the life of their loved one. Seropositive wives' experiences revolved around the core themes of preserving the family and learning whom to count on.

Participant narratives highlight that care receiving constitutes a unique life world. Going beyond the passive acceptance of support, care receiving embraces a multidimensional experience, enmeshed inextricably with the incumbent's developmental stage and gender, and with the psychosocial character of the illness—in this case, its stigmatising, terminal and progressively debilitating nature. The reassurance of being cared for and supported rests uneasily against the shame of being dependent, creating an approach-avoidance conflict. Yet, HIV-infected people's receipt of positive support has been found to go a long way in helping them to cope with their experiences, maintain their health and delay illness progression (Bisset and Gray 1994; Green 1994; Kadushin 1996; Rawat 1999; Thomson 1994). More recently, Bastardo and Kimberlin (2000) have shown a significant positive relation between health-related quality of life (HRQL) and social support in seropositive individuals in Venezuela. Emotional support correlated highest with HRQL measures. Receipt of, and satisfaction with, social support has been found to facilitate healthy and adaptive coping in seropositive people (Leserman et al. 1992). Recent studies in psychoneuroimmunology have shown that self reported social support is significant to the prediction of progression of the immune function, though the significance of social support in regard to the mortality rate remains to be established. Moreover, psychological reactions also influence immune system functioning (Theorell et al. 1995). Counselling positive people about the benefits of support for their health maintenance assumes significance not only in order to ease the process of care receiving, but also to reduce negative feelings associated with the dependence status, which in their own right are known to have adverse consequences for disease progression.

Male care receivers' emotional reactions to the terminal diagnosis point out to a life change event. As Millon et al. (1989) and Teguis and Ahmed (1992) point out, the shadow of death looming over the individual engenders a reexamination of his/her perception and philosophy of life. With HIV, a person can no longer take life for granted. Basic questions about one's ideological approach to life are raised, resulting in reprioritising needs, desires and responsibilities in order to make the most of the time left. Many seropositive people say that though it was unfortunate that an HIV diagnosis provided an impetus for change, the resultant life modifications have prompted fulfilling and rewarding experiences. Since positive individuals confront tasks usually relegated to one's final ageing years when the dying trajectory is more expected and for which people are gradually prepared, AIDS symbolises a sudden death, with positive individuals required to complete tasks not typically experienced at their age (Millon et al. 1989; Teguis and Ahmed 1992). Programmes of emotional support including counselling, support groups and self-help groups, which facilitate working through the emotional turmoil and which help seropositive individuals utilise their time optimally, and so restore their well-being and fulfilment in the post-diagnosis phase, are relevant, given the sense of loss participants report. Shaw (1992), Teguis (1992) and Teguis and Ahmed (1992) list the various losses of the seropositive individual: loss of finances, job, or healthcare security; stigmatisation and social ostracism; loss of pride and self-esteem; loss of a sense of stability, control and concreteness; loss of future hopes, dreams and goals; loss of one's entire peer group; multiple death losses and traumatic degenerative ones; loss of youth, vigour, physical appearance, energy; loss of opportunity to marry and form a family; loss of relationships, especially intimate ones; loss of confidence, sense of reality or perspective about what might constitute adequate coping; loss of self-image/self-worth, attractiveness/livability/special qualities; and loss of sexual interest. Glover and Miller (1990) point out that these losses give rise to emotions that are intense, explosive and recurrent. Working through the enormous tragedy posed by HIV is important, not only to come to terms with the experience and to maintain the optimistic outlook required for longevity and quality of emotional life, but also to find the fortitude to make the most of the time available and to complete unfinished business, if possible, and to see to practical matters. Successfully coming through the challenge usually gives rise to spiritual insight and wisdom that come at the end of a long life (Griffin 1992). The role of emotional support services outlined earlier in such endeavours cannot be undermined. To this end, interventions with the positive person's family or support network may also be relevant since the process of resolution could be affected by their conspiracy of silence/denial and by their reluctance to confront various issues, as if by doing so, their reality can be diminished (Lippmann et al. 1993; O'Donnell 1992).

Caregivers' interpretation of their role as an attempt to extend the life of their care receiver adds a new dimension to our understanding, suggesting that illness outcome is significant in the construction of caregiver role identity. For caregivers, following the knowledge of the fatality of HIV infection, caregiving was not just about role performance/tasks/responsibilities, but went beyond behaviours and actions to embody deeply cherished sentiments and intensely private meanings which symbolised the value attached to the care receiver. These sentiments and meanings served as the underlying motivation for caregiving, and helped caregivers to either overcome or obliterate their experience of burden and transcend their negative reactions to the source of the infection. More empirical research to establish the influence of terminal prognoses in the caregiving trajectory across a range of illnesses, is required for a deeper appreciation of this finding. Emotional support programmes, such as individual and group counselling and therapies, to help caregivers work through the affective reactions to the positive diagnosis, are recommended.

Wives' perceptions of their experiences fit in with the matrix in which Indian tradition and culture define women. That is, a woman's identity is wholly outlined by her relationships with others; as obedient daughter, faithful wife (and daughter-in-law); nurturant mother (more particularly of sons); as the all powerful mother-in-law and then the benevolent grandmother (Bhogle 1999). Srinivas (1978) remarks that Indian culture has venerated the woman in all the roles that she plays. She is rarely praised for being a woman in her own right, but is always understood and explained in terms of others. Her feminine qualities of fidelity, chastity, gentleness and nurturance are valued, and from later childhood, there is a deliberate attempt to train and mould girls into 'good' women, who are docile, submissive and self-effacing (Bhogle 1999). Being a good woman necessarily means regarding the husband as a god, even if he is useless and seeks pleasure elsewhere (Kakar 1988), as institutionalised in the concept of *pativrata* (Chitnis 1988). Restraining their sexuality while their husbands are allowed sexual freedom before and after marriage forms an important component (Ramasubban 1995). Yet, the process of socialising girls is done with a special kind of lenient affection and compassion, because families are aware that daughters are with them for a short period and that when they go to their in-law families, they are most likely to face hostility and even rejection. It is, therefore, taken for granted that while a girl is being socialised for her adult roles, and this is done with considerable discipline and strictness in the natal home, she is simultaneously treated with love and indulgence as her natal family members know that they will inevitably have to lose her to an uncertain future. Natal families' positive and protective responses towards married daughters are extensions of their affection for the latter in the pre-marital days (Kakar 1988). The unsupportive behaviour of the in-law family and the women's hesitation to solicit support from the natal family are also linked to their status in society. Though women's devotion to their husbands is expected to be extended to the husbands' families, and they upon marriage are expected to renounce their natal families and become integrated into their in-law families (ibid.), the latter families do not always completely accept their daughters-in-law. Most often, particularly in the early years, the women are treated as outsiders, and blamed and ill-treated for any mishap. Yet, whatever be her in-laws and her husband, a woman knows that there is no going back home for her (ibid.). Under such stringent social conditions, it is hardly surprising that women do not wish to be found wanting in their caregiving. Any lapse on their part blemishes their reputations and invites criticisms about their natal family's regard for cultural traditions and process of socialisation.

Women's roles revolve around what feminist economists term as 'caring labour', which includes child care, elder care and all the invisible work that goes into making the home a place of comfort, and which is generally undertaken at considerable economic costs to themselves, with implications for achieving gender equality (Agarwal 2000). Indeed, women's assumption of the earner role is also part of their caring labour repertoire because it arises from their positions as flexible household resources (Banerjee 1999), which dictate that they undertake whatever task is necessary (including entry into the public sphere of paid employment), to bail the family out of crises.

Agarwal (2000) cites various viewpoints to explain what causes women to undertake caring labour. One view, put forward by Amartya Sen, but also widely shared, is that in 'traditional societies' such as India, women may tend to lack a clear perception of individual self-interest; that they may suffer from a form of false consciousness in that they value family well-being more than their own. Other scholars argue that women are by nature more altruistic than men and derive pleasure out of providing caring labour; or that they have a less 'separatist' self, or are socialised so as to sacrifice their own well-being for those of their children. According to Agarwal, both versions of the idea that motivations are gendered in this way are interesting but debatable. For example, with regard to false consciousness, it is difficult to infer from people's observable behaviour whether they conform to an unequal social order because they accept its legitimacy, or because they lack options. The overt appearance of compliance, therefore, does not necessarily mean that women lack perception of their best interests. It could indicate a survival strategy that arises from their constraints (such as lack of money) to pursue their interests. Compliance need not imply complicity. The idea that women are more inclined towards altruism than men is equally debatable, although unlike the notion of false perception, altruism implies self-awareness. Some women's observed actions suggest that they are more altruistic than men. For example, poor women typically spend their earnings on family needs. In many Indian families, women also eat last and feed the best food to their sons and husbands. However, this could stem from self-interest. With limited outside options, women might seek to maximise family welfare because it is in their long-term self-interest (even if it reduces their immediate well-being), insofar as women are more socially and economically dependent on the family than are men, and this dependence is longer lasting since, on an average, they have higher life expectancies (ibid.). Moreover, since women's social status in adulthood is tied to marriage and motherhood, they derive their positions from their husbands, and hence express apprehensions over possible widowhood, since it makes them vulnerable on various fronts (D'Cruz and Bharat 2001a). Agarwal (2000) thus argues that if women with weak social and resource positions expend their energies and earnings on the family, this is as consistent with self-interest as it is with altruism. Agarwal concludes by stating that basically, most Indian women are likely to accept the substantial burden of domestic work and child care because they lack alternatives outside marriage and feel a sense of responsibility, which Folbre (in ibid.) terms as socially-imposed altruism. Women often view such responsibilities as a form of social duress, and express this sometimes with resignation and at other times with bitterness (ibid.).

The findings of the study have implications for intervention. Yet, to be effective, intervention should not be restricted to the level of women only. Women's experiences are contextualised in the larger society of which they form a part. Bringing about a change for women necessitates working at all levels that impinge upon women's experiences.

At the larger societal level, changes in the social structure are required that would alter the inferior status accorded to women. Real empowerment requires long-term solutions such as changing paternalistic institutions and ending women's economic dependence on men. For women to become truly empowered, occupational segregation and feminisation of poverty must cease. Women must also acquire greater control over their bodies as well as a women-centred concept of sexuality. Control of the heterosexual epidemic calls for a close look at gender role socialisation—not just of women's roles but also of men's roles (Campbell 1999). In the Indian context, though there are many legal, constitutional and policy-level protections and opportunities for women (Chitnis 1988), they have not translated into attitudinal and value changes and hence, have made little difference to the status of women.

Specific to HIV/AIDS, given the predominance of heterosexual transmission in India, prevention efforts need to take into account power relations based on gender. Interventions are generally gender neutral, assuming that gender roles are static and failing to take into account the socialisation process that increases women's risk of contracting the HIV infection. Interventions need to be gender specific, recognising women's 'permanent inequality' (Miller in Sherr 1993) in status and power. Planners need to recognise that the risks involved in initiating HIV risk reduction changes in intimate relationships is greater for women than for men. This is so because as per a woman's identity, sex is something she gives to a man, and so safer sex negotiations require her to step out of her assigned role and potentially engage in conflict with men. Traditionally, women are expected to be submissive, passive, docile and dependent. However, HIV prevention requires women to be assertive in negotiating safer sex, and this goes contrary to their socialisation. As a result of the unequal social statuses of women and men, negotiations between them for safer sex are more complex than if they had been equals. For those women who are dependent on men for economic and social support, the ways by which they can reduce their risk of HIV infection may be limited. Thus, prevention efforts that educate women, but require behavioural changes by their male sex partners, may not work. For example, women may know of the benefits of using condoms but may not be able to convince their male partners to do so (Campbell 1999). Gorna (1996) maintains that mutual monogamy is not a viable option for women because of gender power differentials—that is, their partners may not be monogamous. Thus, mutual monogamy is actually quite dangerous. Many women subscribe to it with tragic results if their partners do not. According to her, 80 per cent of women become infected from their one and only partner.

Women's needs for support must be addressed adequately and comprehensively. The provision of emotional support, respite care, material and financial assistance, support with regard to treatment and shelter and planning for the future, employment and training, help with caregiving (especially if earning is an unavoidable role for women), and attention to health needs (especially those of seropositive women), are of utmost importance. Programmes that assist with child care while women work and seek treatment are also imperative.

Women and their natal families need to be made more aware of the former's rights in the matrimonial home. In-law families must be sensitised not only to the predicament of their caregiving daughters-in-law, especially those who are seropositive, but must be also made aware of the latter's rights. Long-standing cultural beliefs need to be challenged, and a different world view presented.

Avenues for legal redress in case of violation of women's rights, and awareness of these avenues, are also called for. Such services should be provided through developmental programmes for women as well as through supportive services in the field of HIV/AIDS.

Further research on the experiences of seropositive women must centre attention on women outside the marital union including single women, those in commercial sex work and those in non-legal relationships. Given the position of women in Indian society and the moral stigma attached to HIV/AIDS, it would be worthwhile to systematically study the experiences of these women, particularly in reference to the various modes of the HIV infection and to compare their predicament to that of their married and divorced sisters. The utility of this work would lie in its identification of areas of action for them.

An important finding emerging from the study that adds on to our understanding of the experiences of elderly caregivers, is the role of power relationships in the family stemming from control over economic resources. Though tradition dictates awe and respect for elders in the family and community, current changes in social values such as growing individualism and consumerism, urbanisation and westernisation, changes in the status and self-perceptions of women, women's employment and the economic dependence status of many old people in the absence of social security, are altering the ways in which elderly people are being perceived (Shagle 1995). Shah (1999) maintains that the attitudes and sentiments with which elderly people are regarded and treated determines the quality of their lives. Where they are cherished and considered to be integral parts of the family, they enjoy a happy and valued existence. However, where elderly people are seen as liabilities because of their physical or economic dependence or both, abuse in various forms and degrees is sometimes manifest. Desai and Naik (1982) state that where old age is seen as bringing a dramatic shift in power and authority, especially in cases of economic dependence, influence on family decisions is drastically reduced and participation in family life curtailed. This is true even in cases where elderly family members are assisting with various household functions such as the care of grandchildren, management of daily domestic chores and so on, when their children or children-in-law are engaged in outside employment. As D'Cruz (1998) notes, in contemporary society, elders in the family, being considered redundant and parasitic on family resources, may be subject to various brutalities such as physical neglect and emotional abuse, while simultaneously being used to perform various household tasks without being given due respect. For elderly caregivers in such circumstances, the process of providing care which is already fraught with various challenges not only becomes more difficult, but also dissatisfying because of restrictions on care provision. The issue of caregiver health status in the case of elderly caregivers is also relevant. Undoubtedly, elderly caregivers constitute a special group with a unique set of concerns that must be recognised and addressed by policy makers and service providers. Within the group of elderly caregivers, research attention to grandparent caregivers is needed, given their high incidence in the context of HIV/AIDS.

There is also a growing recognition of the role of children as caregivers. Though the present inquiry has thrown some light on their experiences via the narrative of a seropositive woman, no empirical investigation focusing exclusively on the lives of this group of caregivers has been undertaken in India. Given the fact that the number of child caregivers in India is expected to rise, their contribution to family care in HIV/AIDS cannot be ignored, nor can their experiences and needs. However, insufficient documentation impedes an appropriate response to their situation. Based on our current knowledge, child caregivers need emotional, physical, financial and material support. The initiation of programmes where volunteers from the community or professionals/paraprofessionals from healthcare agencies share some of these children's tasks, providing respite care, is of relevance and could help children to attend school, socialise and experience at least a part of their childhood. Research in this area will be useful in enhancing the efficacy of programmes and policies.

The literature on HIV/AIDS includes information on seropositive caregivers such as wives, mothers, children and gay men. However, in the Indian context, these data are available essentially for wives, as this study as well as earlier works such as Bharat (1996) and D'Cruz (2003a) point out. A complete picture of the dynamics of family care in HIV/AIDS would be possible only if all seropositive caregiving groups were included. The emergent information would facilitate appropriate intervention that would target each group's particular needs and concerns.

Though the research included quasi-family contexts, it was able to provide only a limited view of the caregiving and care receiving experiences of marginalised groups such as eunuchs, CSWs, IVDUs, homosexuals, and those living in unconventional families, such as those living by themselves in single member households. Conducting a study to understand their experiences and needs would be valuable. This would not only provide information on the spectrum of caregiver and care receiver experiences in HIV/AIDS, but also serve as a basis for appropriate policy and programme planning in relation to marginalised populations.

Insights into the caregiver–care receiver relationship have emerged essentially from work on Alzheimer's dementia (AD), where primarily cognitive changes in the care receiver are responsible for the evolving relationship. In HIV/AIDS, relational changes reflect greater causal complexity being determined by the nature of care received, the perception of the source of the infection and the ability to transcend negative feelings related to this, the presence of reciprocity (even in emotional terms of thoughtfulness and sensitivity), and the extent of obligation in the relationship. While the caregiver–care receiver relationship in the context of HIV/AIDS is little understood so far, some of the factors referred to above have been cited in literature describing family relationships following a seropositive diagnosis. Glover and Miller (1990), for example, maintain that HIV/AIDS tips the balance in family relationships and becomes the only significant factor in decision making in the family. According to Bharat (1996) and Lippmann et al. (1993), the quality of pre-morbid family ties and the perception of the source of infection are decisive factors. Understanding the dynamics of caregiver–care receiver relations and applying insights here to strengthen connectedness in the dyad are important agendas, since as Himmelweit (1999) points out, caregiver–care receiver interactions are inextricably linked with the process(es) of caregiving (and care receiving). Working with caregivers and family members to resolve their negative feelings about the source of HIV infection assumes priority, given its influence on the caregiving process. As a part of this, elucidating to families the relevance of support in stalling the progress of the infection would be useful. Similarly, sensitising care receivers to the experiences of their caregivers could result in gestures of emotional reciprocation on their part, which add to caregivers' well-being and, in turn, to the caregiver-care receiver relationship.

The stigma associated with HIV/AIDS and its implications for caregiving and care receiving were highlighted by participants in numerous ways, lending support to earlier literature. Enacted stigma in the social network, at the workplace and during health seeking, was reported. Perceived stigma was so strong that it complicated decisions involving disclosure even in 'innocent' cases, and hampered need fulfilment and support seeking. Crocker and Quinn (2001), reviewing literature on stigma, point out that a stigmatised person is one whose social identity or membership in a social category calls into question his or her full humanity—the person is flawed, devalued or spoiled in the eyes of others. Stigmatised individuals are often the targets of negative stereotypes and elicit emotional reactions such as pity, anger, anxiety or disgust. The central feature of stigma, however, is the devaluation and dehumanisation by others. Herek (n.d.) and Herek and Mitnick (1996) define AIDS-related stigma as prejudice, discounting, discrediting and discrimination, directed at people perceived to have HIV/AIDS, and at the individuals, groups and communities with which they are associated. The primary targets of AIDS stigma are individuals with HIV and those who are perceived to be HIV-infected. Secondary targets of AIDS stigma are positive people's partners, family members and loved ones, as well as professionals and volunteers who work with them, all of whom experience what is termed as a courtesy stigma, to use Goffman's term. Secondary targets also include uninfected members of groups popularly perceived as linked to the AIDS epidemic. Perpetrators of AIDS stigma derive their negative reactions from two fundamental sources: instrumental stigma which refers to outcomes directly related to HIV, such as its degenerative, fatal and transmissible nature; and symbolic stigma, which arises from the social meanings attached to the infection, linked essentially to the groups associated with it and behaviours that transmit it and which result in the perception of positive people as an outgroup (Herek n.d.; Herek and Mitnick 1996).

AIDS stigma is widely recognised as a problem that not only hampers care and support, as we have seen in this study, but also interferes with prevention. Fear of stigma, for example, impedes disclosure of serostatus even to sexual partners, which interferes with risk reduction. It also deters people at risk for HIV from being tested and from seeking information and assistance with risk reduction. The politics of AIDS stigma hinders societal responses to the epidemic. The media were initially slow to cover the disease because of its prevalence among stigmatised groups. Stigma permeated the immediate legislative responses of many countries, and extensive resources that might have otherwise gone to prevention have been used to respond to punitive AIDS legislation. On account of stigma, AIDS educators have been reluctant to provide clear and explicit risk reduction information to individuals at risk. Since stigma hampers society's ability to respond effectively to HIV/AIDS, counteracting it remains a critical public health objective. However, effective intervention here has to be preceded by extensive social and behavioural studies on the cultural context and manifestations of stigma, the targets of stigma and the perpetrators of stigma, so that we may fully understand this multi-faceted concept. Such research must take into account the evolving epidemic which brings with it changes in the nature of AIDS stigma. Knowledge thus generated will be critical for governments and health providers, as they debate policies and strategies to combat AIDS stigma and manage HIV treatment, care and prevention (Herek and Mitnick 1996).

Meanwhile, organising and implementing HIV/AIDS awareness programmes in the community would have advantages. Being armed with information about the infection, members of the community would not only refrain from behaviours that transmit the virus, but also dismiss myths and misconceptions. Moreover, they would be sensitised to the experiences that seropositive individuals, their caregivers and their families undergo, and instead of discriminating against them, they would reach out to them in supportive ways. Through the creation of community support systems, positive people, their caregivers and their families, being reassured of an understanding response, would come forward and seek assistance. Educating HIV-infected individuals, their caregivers and their families about their rights, and about opportunities for redressal in the event of their violation, is an important agenda.

Equally important is the need for work organisations to develop humanistic policies on HIV/AIDS. These policies ensure the welfare and protection of the seropositive individual and are openly committed to viewing HIV/AIDS within the workplace in terms of social justice and human dignity. Although allowing for the differentiation of individuals with HIV/AIDS where necessary, this is done in a manner which is explicitly non-exclusionary and which guarantees protection if required. The attempt is to normalise AIDS, to treat it as 'just another disease', as a means of pre-empting a homophobic attack. Such normalisation is in contrast with defensive policies, which are better understood in terms of 'abnormalisation', to the extent that they emphasise the difference/'otherness'/threatening quality of AIDS per se, and in doing so, reinforce the 'myth of otherness' and danger which has been attached to those groups who are directly affected. Defensive policies have a high degree of both conditionality and exclusion and retain the maximum room for legal manoeuvre for the organisation and the protection of its interests, often at the expense, ultimately, of those with HIV/AIDS. An empowering organisational response that offers the prospect of dealing constructively with the practical, medical workplace needs of people with HIV/AIDS, while at the same time providing a separate and comprehensive commitment to equal opportunities based on minority rights per se, would be ideal (Goss and Adam-Smith 1994).

Participant narratives of discrimination within the healthcare system add on to documented instances of enacted stigma while seeking healthcare, reported from across the globe. Barbour (1994); Bharat (1999); Grunseit and Kippax (1992); Hackl et al. (1997); McCann (1999); Sathiamoorthy and Solomon (1997); Sewpaul and Mahlalela (1998); Stein et al. (1997) and Thomson (1994), assert that discriminatory responses from healthcare workers are common and include refusal to admit and treat, breach of confidentiality, testing without consent, neglect of patients, insensitive and judgemental responses, displaying negative attitudes, warning other staff of the potential risk or danger of HIV, taking additional precautions or avoiding working with identified patients. It is believed that these arise due to homophobia, condemnation of prostitution and injecting drug use, and concern about contagion (McCann 1999). Such responses impinge on the infected individual's overall experience of HIV, and on the experience of care and support in particular. McCann's study examines why some doctors and nurses are reluctant to deal with HIV-positive people. The four main themes which emerged from his study were perceptions about sexual promiscuity, blaming certain patients with HIV/AIDS, belief in the right to refuse to provide care, and discriminatory care and treatment (ibid.). It is also possible that lack of training and supervision of healthcare professionals impedes their role enactment (Stein et al. 1997). Barbour (1994) and Hackl et al.'s (1997) prediction that the healthcare system and its workers may also be responsible for breaking the confidentiality of a patient's diagnosis and for indiscriminate disclosure either directly or indirectly, which in turn make the HIV-infected person vulnerable to the spread of the diagnosis and to stigma and discrimination from healthcare workers, other patients and people from their social networks, was borne out in the study.

The experience of discrimination has been found to create severe psychological distress for seropositive people and their families, precipitating feelings of loneliness at a very trying and difficult period. Indeed, the perception of being unsupported has implications for illness progression as various inquiries have shown.

Since the private sector is increasingly becoming a major component of India's healthcare system, and the public sector, on the other hand, is turned to for free treatment and hospitalisation, considering including them as components of HIV/AIDS-related service organisations appears practical. Undoubtedly, given their attitudes towards HIV/AIDS, such a task is a herculean one. A comprehensive and large inquiry, building on the work of Bharat (1999), into the attitudes of the private and public health sectors towards HIV/AIDS, and the reasons behind their refusal to treat seropositive individuals, would be useful in understanding the motives behind their actions. Within this endeavour, research into the behaviour of different categories of healthcare personnel, in both these sectors, should be incorporated, with a view to ascertaining the factors underlying their actions in the context of HIV/AIDS. Based on such data, attempts to secure their participation in HIV/AIDS care can be worked out.

While support from healthcare workers was limited, its location largely within the voluntary sector confirms Altman's (1994) and New et al.'s (1998) idea that community-based responses have been the main means to deal with the crisis of HIV/AIDS and have played pivotal roles in leading the way. Recognition of the contribution and commitment of the voluntary sector should not deflect attention away from the shortcomings in the healthcare system as a whole. Indeed, inadequacies in India's healthcare system in terms of policy, plan and programme focus, resource allocation, sector-wise performance, geographical distribution of services, manpower imbalances, quality of facilities and so on, have been extensively documented (see D'Cruz and Bharat 2001b for a comprehensive review). These are expected to worsen with the structural adjustment programme (SAP) (Qadeer 2000). This programme, introduced by the World Bank to help the health sector sustain itself, includes cuts in public spending for health services and shifts to strengthen population control; shifting curative care to the private sector; introduction of cost recovery mechanisms in private hospitals as well as all sources of financing, such as user fees, insurance, self/community financing; defining essential clinical and public health packages; and tackling poverty through SAP, education and women's employment (World Bank 1993).

Indeed, the work of the voluntary sector in HIV/AIDS should be seen in the light of the SAP which promotes cuts in social sector expenditure and policies of community care. That the government has used the laudable role of NGOs to its advantage by formally placing the onus of care and support on the family and on the voluntary sector through the adoption of the continuum of care approach in HIV/AIDS, cannot be disputed (NACO 1998; Sethi 1999; Yaima et al. 1997). In this way, the basic responsibility for care has been put on to the family, and on to NGOs who support them in this role. However, is an exclusive reliance on families and NGOs a viable solution? Bharat (1996) and D'Cruz (2003a) have convincingly demonstrated the negative impact of HIV/AIDS on the family economy which unleashes deprivation for the entire household, as well as the burden on women who, as society's traditional caregivers and households' flexible labour resource, have to provide care and support to not just their seropositive relative, but also to other family members. A complete drain of emotional, physical, material and financial resources is reported by such families, not to mention the alienation from the social network due to the stigmatising nature of the virus. While the strengths of NGOs are derived from their grassroot approach, small size, low operating costs, dedicated leadership, professionalism, flexibility and responsiveness, their shortcomings include uncertainty over finance, limited area of coverage, isolationism, difficulty in replicating their endeavours (Chatterjee 1988; Smith 1989) and collapse of a programme following their exit from an area (Bhatia 1993). Weighing their pros and cons, Chatterjee (1988: 143) considers them to be 'little pockets of excellence which do not carry much significance', and which reach less than 5 per cent of the poor (Chatterjee 1993). Yet, given their exemplary contribution in the context of HIV/AIDS, it would be of relevance to replicate their strengths within the entire healthcare system, so that beneficiaries may be better served and variation in available facilities may be reduced. Baseline data, through a critical examination of the functioning of these voluntary agencies, the services they provide, their ideologies, organisational patterns, and strengths and weaknesses, need to be generated prior to conceptualising and executing this venture.

Overall, stepping up secondary- and tertiary-level medical and supportive services, including emotional, material and financial support, and counselling services, in the public, private and voluntary sectors, for caregivers, care receivers and their families, is the need of the hour. A greater number of services, covering a greater range of needs, and more beneficiaries, is called for. Supportive services take on greater significance in the light of HIV's stigmatising nature, which creates isolation and hampers support seeking and need fulfilment.

There is an urgent need to regulate the public and private healthcare systems to make them accountable and to ensure the quality of care that they provide. Mechanisms in this direction would eliminate discrimination and violation of ethical guidelines, develop atmospheres of support for patients and their families, as well as improve facilities and services. An important step here is educating healthcare workers about the pandemic. Such a move would dispel myths and misconceptions about HIV/AIDS existing in the minds of healthcare workers, lower the chances of them practising stigmatising behaviour, and enhance the likelihood of them providing quality care, treatment and support. Avenues for redressal in the event of violation of positive peoples' rights and of stigma and discrimination should be created. Additionally, raising healthcare standards so that interventions here do not result in the transmission of the HIV infection, cannot be postponed.

Apart from the limited support provided by the healthcare system, the absence of a caregiver and a family focus here is also a matter of significant concern, given the onus of responsibility and degree of burden on them. Yet, this is not a new finding in the Indian context, particularly in the case of physical illness (see D'Cruz 2003b for a review). In the West, the family focus in health and illness interventions is being stressed, in recognition of the unit's pivotal role. That is, families are seen as the primary context of care, as the social group most affected by illness, as determinants of health and illness, and as allies in treatment. In response, strategies such as family medicine, family therapy/counselling and family social work are employed (D'Cruz 2003b). A similar approach is called for in the Indian context to assist caregivers and caregiving families. Interventions for caregivers including counselling services, support programmes, respite care facilities and support groups, which would facilitate role performance and management of burden and emotional distress, should be given priority. Within these, special programmes catering to the needs of seropositive caregivers, women caregivers, elderly caregivers, child caregivers, caregivers of positive people with multiple chronic conditions, and caregivers in households with multiple seropositive members, must be devised.

Institutionalisation as a means of care runs contrary to policies of community care, but is seen as an important alternative for those who have no blood/marital families to look after them or who have been rejected by their families. It is also greatly appreciated by family caregivers as a source of respite and of protection against (seemingly) contagious opportunistic infections. Besides these issues, given the psychosocial features of the HIV infection, namely, its gradual onset, long-drawn course, terminal prognosis and incapacitating outcome, which underscore the length of time over which care is needed and the progressively demanding tasks involved (both of which can sometimes overwhelm caregivers and families), can we eliminate institutionalisation altogether? What alternatives can we develop to provide sustained, positive support? Addressing these issues is an important priority for policy makers and service providers working in the field of HIV/AIDS.

The concern of most participants about their inability to avail of highly active anti-retroviral treatment (HAART) because of its exorbitant cost, came out clearly in the study. At the time when data were collected for this inquiry, the reduced price of anti-retrovirals, as currently available in India thanks to the efforts of the pharmaceutical company Cipla, was not yet a reality (Ghangurde 2000). While a few participants had turned to alternative systems of medicine and spoke of their benefits, further research is needed to conclusively prove their efficacy. Moreover, the range of alternatives available here includes those rooted in traditionally accepted systems, such as Ayurveda and Homoeopathy, as well as in unscientific versions, practised by quacks. Patients need to be aware of all these complexities and must be cautioned against blindly believing widespread messages promoting these regimens, without cross-checking their basis. This would help them guard against harmful medications and excessive expenditure. It is also important for a body to be created to monitor treatment programmes on various grounds, such as their proven basis, whether they are currently under trial without the knowledge of the positive people using them, whether the positive people undergoing the treatment are unknowingly being used in the trials, and so on. Overall, across allopathic and alternative systems, costs of treatment (both direct and indirect) need to be re-examined, notwithstanding national and international economic compulsions, and attempts to reduce costs and subsidise treatments must be made.

The world over, as families shoulder the responsibility of providing care to their seropositive loved ones, McGrath et al. (1994) warn that in the absence of adequate support, families will be unable to cope. According to them, the loss of equilibrium could precipitate a sense of disintegration, which in turn could call into question the future of the family as an institution.

References

Abel, E.K. (1991). *Who care for the elderly? Public policy and the experience of adult daughters.* Philadelphia: Temple University Press.

Agarwal, B. (2000). The idea of gender equality. In R. Thapar (ed.), *India: Another millennium,* pp. 36–65. New Delhi: Viking.

Aggarwal, O.P., Sharma, A.K. and Indrayan, A. (1997). *HIV/AIDS research in India.* New Delhi: NACO.

Aldous, J. (1994). 'Someone to watch over me: Family responsibilities and their realisation across family lives'. In E. Kahana, D.E. Biegel and M.L. Winkle (eds), *Family caregiving across the lifespan,* pp. 42–68. California: Sage.

Altman, D. (1994). *Power and community.* London: Taylor & Francis.

Ankrah, E.M. (1994). 'The impact of HIV/AIDS on the family and other significant relationships: The African clan revisited'. In R. Bor and J. Elford (eds), *The family and HIV,* pp. 23–44. London: Cassell.

Archbold, P.G. (1991). 'Distinguished research lectureship: An interdisciplinary approach to family caregiving research'. *Communicating Nursing Research* 24: 27–42.

Archbold, P.G., Stewart, B.J., Greenlick, M. and Harvath, T. (1990). 'Mutuality and preparedness as predictors of caregiver role strain'. *Research in Nursing and Health* 13: 375–84.

Aronson, J. (1992). 'Women's sense of responsibility for the care of old people: "But who else is going to do it?"'. *Gender and Society* 6: 8–29.

Asthana, S. (1996). 'AIDS-related policies, legislation and programme implementation in India'. *Health Policy and Planning* 11: 184–97.

Banerjee, N. (1999). 'Household dynamics and women in a changing economy'. In M. Krishnaraj, R.M. Sudarshan and A. Shariff (eds), *Gender, population and development,* pp. 245–66. Delhi: Oxford University Press.

Barber, C.E., Fisher, B.L. and Pasley, K. (1990). 'Family care of Alzheimer's disease patients: Predictors of subjective and objective burden'. *Family Perspective* 24: 289–309.

Barbour, R.S. (1994). 'A telling tale: AIDS workers and confidentiality'. In P. Aggleton, P. Davies and G. Hart (eds), *AIDS: Foundations for the future.* London: Taylor & Francis.

Barlow, J. (1994). 'Social issues: An overview'. In J. Bury (ed.), *Working with women and AIDS.* London: Routledge.

Bastardo, Y.M. and Kimberlin, C.L. (2000). 'Relationship between quality of life, social support and disease related factors in HIV infected persons in Venezuela'. *AIDS Care* 12: 673–84.

Bengston, V.L. and Roberts, R.E. (1991). 'Intergenerational solidarity in aging families'. *Journal of Marriage and the Family* 53: 856–70.

Berg-Weger, M., McGartland Rubio, D. and Tebb, S.S. (2000). 'Depression as a mediator: Viewing caregiver well-being and strain in a different light'. *Families in Society* 8: 162–73.

Bharat, S. (1995). 'HIV/AIDS and the family: Issues in care and support'. *Indian Journal of Social Work* 56: 177–94.

————. (1996). *Facing the challenge: Household and community responses to HIV/AIDS in Mumbai, India.* Project report. Mumbai: TISS.

————. (1999). *HIV/AIDS related discrimination, stigmatisation and denial in India (A study in Mumbai and Bangalore).* Project report. Mumbai: TISS.

Bharat, S. and Aggleton, P. (1999). 'Facing the challenge: Household responses to HIV/AIDS in Mumbai, India'. *AIDS Care* 11: 31–44.

Bhatia, K. (1993). 'The NGO movement in health'. In N.H. Antia and K. Bhatia (eds), *People's health in people's hands*, pp. 75–85. Bombay: FRCH.

Bhogle, S. (1999). 'Gender roles: The construct in the Indian context'. In T.S. Saraswathi (ed.), *Culture, socialisation and human development*, pp. 278–300. New Delhi: Sage.

Bishop, A. and Scudder, J. (1991). *Nursing: The practice of caring.* New York: National League for Nursing Press.

Bisset, K. and Gray, J. (1994). 'Feelings and needs of women who are HIV positive'. In J. Bury (ed.), *Working with women and AIDS.* London: Routledge.

Blackburn, J. (1988). 'Chronic health problems of the elderly'. In C.S.Chilman, E.N. Nunally and F.M. Cox (eds), *Chronic illness and disability*, pp. 108–22. California: Sage.

Blieszner, R. and Shifflett, P.A. (1990). 'The effects of Alzheimer's disease on close relationships between patients and caregivers'. *Family Relations* 39: 57–62.

Bombay Metropolitan Region Development Authority/BMRDA. (1995). *Draft regional plan for Bombay Metropolitan Region, 1996–2011.* Mumbai: BMRDA.

Boss, P., Caron, W., Horbal, G. and Mortimer, G. (1990). 'Predictors of depression in caregivers of dementia patients: Boundary ambiguity and mastery'. *Family Process* 29: 245–54.

Bowers, B. (1988). 'Family perceptions of care in a nursing home'. *The Gerontologist* 38: 261–368.

Braithwaite, V. (1992). 'Caregiver burden: Making the concept scientifically useful and policy relevant'. *Research on Aging* 14: 3–27.

Brennan, P.F. and Moore, S.M. (1994). 'Caregivers of persons living with AIDS'. In E. Kahana, D.E. Biegel and M.L. Wykle (eds), *Family caregiving across the lifespan*, pp. 159–77. California: Sage.

Brouwer, C.N.M., Lok, C.L., Wolffers, I. and Sebagalls, S. (2000). 'Psychosocial and economic aspects of HIV/AIDS and counselling of caretakers of HIV infected children in Uganda'. *AIDS Care* 12: 535–40.

Brown, M.A. and Stetz, K. (1999). 'The labour of caregiving: A theoretical model of caregiving during potentially fatal illness'. *Qualitative Health Research* 9: 182–97.

Bryman, A. (1988). *Quality and quantity in social research*. London: Unwin Hyman.

Bryman, A. and Burgess, R.G. (1999). 'Qualitative research methodology: A review'. In A. Bryman and R.G. Burgess (eds), *Qualitative research*, Vol. I, pp. ix–xlvi. London: Sage.

Bulger, M.W., Wandersman, A. and Goldman, C.R. (1993). 'Burdens and satisfactions of caregiving: Appraisal of parental care of adults with schizophrenia'. *American Journal of Orthopsychiatry* 63: 255–65.

Burch, R. (1989). 'On phenomenology and its practices'. *Phenomenology + pedagogy* 7: 187–217.

Campbell, C.A. (1999). *Women, families and HIV/AIDS*. New York: Cambridge University Press.

Cancian, F.M. (1987). *Love in America: Gender and self development*. New York: Cambridge University Press.

Cargan, L. and Ballantine, J.H. (2000). *Sociological footprints*. Belmont, CA: Wadsworth.

Carpentier, N., Lesage, A., Goulet, J., Lalonde, P. and Renaud, M. (1992). 'Burden of care for families not living with young schizophrenic relatives'. *Hospital and Community Psychiatry* 43: 38–43.

Cartwright, J.C., Archbold, P.G., Stewart, B.J. and Limandri, B. (1994). 'Enrichment processes in caregiving to frail elders'. *Advances in Nursing Science* 17: 31–43.

Chakrabarti, S., Raj, L., Kulhara, P., Avasthi, A. and Verma, S.K. (1995). 'A comparison of the extent and pattern of family burden in effective disorders and schizophrenia'. *Indian Journal of Psychiatry* 37: 105–12.

Chandrashekhar, C.R., Ranga Rao, N.V.S.S. and Srinivasa Murthy, R. (1991). 'The chronic mentally ill and their families'. In S. Bharat (ed.), *Research on families with problems in India*, Vol. 1. Bombay: TISS.

Chatterjee, M. (1988). *Implementing health policy*. New Delhi: Centre for Policy Research.

————. (1993). 'Health for too many: India's experiments with truth'. In J. Rohde, M. Chatterjee and D. Morley (eds), *Reaching health for all*, pp. 342–77. Delhi: Oxford University Press.

Chesla, C.A. (1991). 'Parents' caring practices with schizophrenic offspring'. *Qualitative Health Research* 1: 446–68.

Chesla, C., Martinson, I. and Muwaswes, M. (1994). 'Continuities and discontinuities in family members' relationships with Alzheimer's patients'. *Family Relations* 43: 3–9.

Chinouya-Mudari, M. and O'Brien, M. (1999). 'African refugee children and HIV/AIDS in London'. In P. Aggleton, G. Hart and P. Davies (eds), *Families and communities responding to AIDS*, pp. 21–34. London: UCL Press.

Chitnis, S. (1988). 'Feminism: Indian ethos and Indian convictions'. In R. Ghadially (ed.), *Women in Indian society*, pp. 81–95. New Delhi: Sage.

Cohen, M.Z. and Omery, A. (1994). 'Schools of phenomenology: Implications for research'. In J.M. Morse (ed.), *Critical issues in qualitative research methods*, pp. 136–57. California: Sage.

Conger, C.O. and Marshall, E.S. (1998). 'Recreating life: Toward a theory of relationship development in acute home care'. *Qualitative Health Research* 8: 526–46.

Cook, J.A. (1988). 'Who "mothers" the chronically mentally ill?'. *Family Relations* 37: 42–49.

Cook, J.A., Hoffschmidt, S., Cohler, B.J. and Pickett, S. (1992). 'Marital satisfaction among parents of the severely mentally ill living in the community'. *American Journal of Orthopsychiatry* 62: 552–63.

Cowles, V.K. and Rodgers, B.L. (1997). 'Struggling to keep on top: Meeting the everyday challenges of AIDS'. *Qualitative Health Research* 7: 98–120.

Creswell, J.W. (1998). *Qualitative inquiry and research design: Choosing among five traditions.* California: Sage.

Crocker, J. and Quinn, D.M. (2001). 'Psychological consequences of devalued identities'. In R. Brown and S.L. Gaertner (eds), *Blackwell handbook of social psychology: Intergroup processes*, pp. 238–60. Massachusetts: Blackwell.

Daly, K. (1992). 'The fit between qualitative research and characteristics of families'. In J.F. Gilgun, K. Daly and G. Handel (eds), *Qualitative methods in family research*, pp. 3–11. Newbury Park: Sage.

D'Cruz, P. (1998). 'The smallest democracy at the heart of society: Myths of the family: Part I'. *Facts Against Myths.* Mumbai: VAK.

——————. (2001). 'Children with HIV/AIDS: Beyond infected and affected'. Paper prepared for UNICEF, on behalf of Committed Communities Development Trust, Mumbai.

——————. (2003a). *In sickness and in health: The family experience of HIV/AIDS in India.* Kolkata: Stree.

——————. (2003b). 'Family focused interventions in health and illness'. *Journal of Health Management* 5: 37–56.

D'Cruz, P. and Bharat, S. (2001a). 'Beyond joint and nuclear: The Indian family revisited'. *Journal of Comparative Family Studies* 32: 167–94.

——————. (2001b). 'Which way to turn: Inadequacies in the health care system in India'. *Journal of Health Management* 3: 85–126.

Denzin, N.K. and Lincoln, Y.S. (1994). 'Introduction: Entering the field of qualitative research'. In N.K. Denzin and Y.S. Lincoln (eds), *Handbook of qualitative research*, pp. 1–19. California: Sage.

Desai, K.G. and Naik, R.D. (1982). 'Problems of retired people in Greater Bombay'. In K.G. Desai (ed.), *Aging in India.* Mumbai: Tata Institute of Social Sciences.

de Bruyn, M., Jackson, H., Wijermars, M., Knight, V.C. and Berkvens, R. (1995). *Facing the challenges of HIV, AIDS, STDs: A gender-based response.* Amsterdam: KIT, Zimbabwe: SAFAIDS, Geneva: WHO.

Dolgin, M. and Phipps, S. (1996). 'Reciprocal influences in family adjustment to childhood cancer'. In L. Baider, C.L. Cooper and A. Kaplan De-Nour (eds), *Cancer and the family*, pp. 73–92. Chichester: John Wiley.

Douglass, L.G. (1997). 'Reciprocal support in the context of cancer: Perspectives of the patient and spouse'. *Oncology Nursing Forum* 24: 1529–36.

Duggal R. (1995). 'Public health budgets: Recent trends'. *Radical Journal of Health (New Series)* 1: 177–82.

Duttmann, A.G. (1996). *At odds with AIDS.* Stanford: Stanford University Press.

Dwyer, J.W. and Coward, R.T. (1992). 'Gender differences in spousal care of impaired elders'. *Family Perspective* 26: 267–80.

Fancey, P. and Keefe, J. (1994). *Annotated bibliography of family interactions with relatives in homes for special care.* Halifax: Nova Scotia Centre on Aging, Mount Saint Vincent.

Feeman, D.J. and Hagen, J.W. (1990). 'Effects of childhood chronic illness on families'. *Social Work in Health Care* 14: 37–53.

Fergus, K.D., Gray, R.E., Fitch, M.I., Labrecque, M. and Phillips, C. (2002). 'Active consideration: Conceptualising patient provided support for spouse caregivers in the context of prostate cancer'. *Qualitative Health Research* 12: 492–514.

Finley, N.J. (1989). 'Theories of family labour as applied to gender difference in caregiving for elderly parents'. *Journal of Marriage and the Family* 51: 79–86.

Forehand, R., Pelton, J., Chance, M., Armistead, L., Morse, E., Morse, P.S. and Stock, M. (1999). 'Orphans of the AIDS epidemic in the United States: Transition-related characteristics and psychosocial adjustment at 6 months after mother's death'. *AIDS Care* 11: 715–22.

Fulks, J.S. and Martin, P. (1993). 'Predictors of active and avoidance coping in family caregivers'. *Family Perspective* 27: 233–49.

Gangakhedkar, R.R., Bentley, M.E., Divekar, A.D., Gadkari, D., Mehendale, S.M., Shepherd, M.E., Bollinger, R.C. and Quinn, T.C. (1997). 'Spread of HIV infection in married monogamous women in India'. *Journal of the American Medical Association* 278: 2090–92.

Garcia, R., de Moya, E.A., Fadul, R., Castellanos, C., Freites, A. and Guerrero, S. (1995). *Household and community responses to HIV/AIDS in the Dominican Republic.* Santo Domingo: Universidad Autonoma De Santo Domingo.

George, L.K. and Gwyther, L.P. (1986). 'Caregiver well-being: A multinational examination of family caregivers of demented adults'. *The Gerontologist* 26: 253–59.

Ghangurde, A. (2000). 'Cipla bags drugs controller approval to manufacture, market anti-AIDS pill'. *Financial Express,* 21 March. Retrieved 14 December 2002 from http://www.financialexpress.com/fe/daily/20000321/fco21025.html

Given, C.W. and Given, B.A. (1994). 'The home care of a patient with cancer: The midlife crisis'. In E. Kahana, D.E. Biegel and M.L. Wykle (eds), *Family caregiving across the life span,* pp. 240–61. California: Sage.

Global Programme on AIDS/GPA. (1995). *1992–93 Progress report: Global programme on AIDS.* Geneva: WHO.

Glover, L. and Miller, D. (1990). 'Counselling in the context of HIV infection & disease'. In A. Mindel (ed.), *AIDS: A pocketbook of diagnosis and management.* Baltimore: Urban & Schwarzenberg.

Goldstein, H. (1990). 'Strength or pathology: Ethical and rhetorical contrasts in approaches to practice'. *Families in Society* 71: 267–75.

Gorna, R. (1996). *Vamps, virgins and victims.* New York: Cassell.

Goss, D. and Adam-Smith, D. (1994). 'Empowerment and disempowerment: The limits and possibilities of workplace policy'. In P. Aggleton, P. Davies and G. Hart (eds), *AIDS: Foundations for the future,* pp. 33–47. London: Taylor & Francis.

Graham, H. (1983). 'Caring: A labour of love'. In J. Finch and D. Groves (eds), *A labor of love: Women, work and caring,* pp. 13–25. London: Routledge & Kegan Paul.

Green, G. (1994). 'Social support and HIV'. In R. Bor and J. Elford (eds), *The family and HIV.* London: Cassell.

Greenberg, J.S., Greenley, J.R., McKee, D., Brown, R. and Griffin-Francell, C. (1993). 'Mothers caring for an adult child with schizophrenia'. *Family Relations* 42: 205–11.

Griffin, R. (1992). 'Living with AIDS: Surviving grief'. In P.I. Ahmed (ed.), *Living and dying with AIDS*, pp. 179–97. New York: Plenum.

Grunseit, A. and Kippax, S. (1992). *Response to HIV/AIDS at the individual, household, community and society levels.* Australia: National Centre for HIV Social Research.

Gupta, I. and Panda, S. (2002). 'The HIV/AIDS epidemic in India: Looking ahead'. In S. Panda, A. Chatterjee and A.S. Abdul-Quader (eds), *Living with the AIDS virus*, pp. 179–96. New Delhi: Sage.

Hackl, K.L., Somlai, A.M., Kelly, J.A. and Kalichman, S.C. (1997). 'Women living with HIV/AIDS: The dual challenge of being a patient and a caregiver'. *Health and Social Work* 22: 53–62.

Haley, W.E. and Pardo, K.M. (1989). 'Relationship of severity of dementia to caregiving stressors'. *Psychology and Aging* 4: 389–92.

Hansen, K., Woelk, G., Jackson, H., Kerkhoven, R., Manjonjori, N., Maramba, P., Mutambirwa, J., Ndimande, E. and Vera, E. (1998). 'The cost of home based care for HIV/AIDS patients in Zimbabwe'. *AIDS Care* 10: 751–59.

Heaphy, B., Weeks, J. and Donovan, C. (1999). 'Narratives of care, love and commitment: AIDS/HIV and non-heterosexual family formations'. In P. Aggleton, P. Davies and G. Hart (eds), *Families and communities responding to AIDS*, pp. 67–82. London: UCL Press.

Heller, T. (1993). 'Aging caregivers of persons with developmental disabilities: Changes in burden placement desire'. In K.A. Roberto (ed.), *The elderly caregiver: Caring for the adults with developmental disabilities*, pp. 21–38. Newbury Park, CA: Sage.

Herek, G.M. (n.d.). *AIDS and stigma.* Retrieved 7 July 2003 from http://psychology.ucdavis.edu/rainbow/html/abs99_intro.pdf

Herek, G.M. and Mitnick, L. (1996). *AIDS and stigma: A conceptual framework and research agenda.* Retrieved 7 July 2003 from http://psychology.ucdavis.edu/rainbow/html/stigma98.pdf

Himmelweit, S. (1999). 'Caring labour'. *The Annals of the American Academy of Political and Social Science,* 561: 27–38.

Hinrichsen, G., Hernandez, N. and Pollack, D. (1992). 'Difficulties and rewards in family care of the depressed older adult'. *The Gerontologist* 32: 486–92.

Hirschfeld, M. (1993). 'Homecare versus institutionalisation: Family caregiving and senile brain disease'. *International Journal of Nursing Studies* 20: 23–32.

Hooyman, N.R. and Gonyea, J. (1995). *Feminist perspectives on family care.* California: Sage.

Horwitz, A.V. (1993). 'Adult siblings as sources of social support for the seriously mentally ill: A test of serial model'. *Journal of Marriage and the Family* 55: 623–32.

Huby, G.O., Teylinger, E.R., Robertson, J.R. and Porter, A.M.D. (1993). 'Community care and community support for women'. In M.A. Johnson and F.D. Johnstone (eds), *HIV infection in women.* London: Churchill Livingstone.

Hull, M.M. (1992). 'Coping strategies of family caregivers in hospice home care'. *Oncology Nursing Forum* 19: 1179–87.

Ingersoll-Dayton, B., Neal, M.B. and Hammer, L.B. (2001). 'Aging parent helping adult children: The experience of the sandwiched generation'. *Family Relations* 50: 262–71.

Jankowski, S., Videka-Sherman, L. and Laquidara-Dickinson, K. (1996). 'Social support networks of confidants to people with AIDS'. *Social Work* 41: 206–13.

Jeon, Y.H. and Madjar, I. (1998). 'Caring for a family member with chronic mental illness'. *Qualitative Health Research* 8: 694–706.

Kadushin, G. (1996). 'Gay men with AIDS and their families of origin: An analysis of social support'. *Health and Social Work* 21: 141–49.

Kahana, E., Kahana, B., Johnson, J.R., Hammond, R.J. and Kercher, K. (1994). 'Developmental changes and family caregiving: Bridging concepts and research'. In E. Kahana, D.E. Biegel and M.L. Wykle (eds), *Family caregiving across the lifespan*, pp. 3–41. California: Sage.

Kakar, S. (1988). 'Feminine identity in India'. In R. Ghadially (ed.), *Women in Indian society*, pp. 44–68. New Delhi: Sage.

Kaye, L.W. and Applegate, J.S. (1990) 'Men as elder caregivers: A response to changing families'. *American Journal of Orthopsychiatry* 60: 86–95.

Kazak, A.E. (1986). 'Families with physically handicapped children'. *Family Process* 25: 265–81.

Kazak, A.E. and Christakis, D.A. (1994). 'Caregiving issues in families of children with chronic medical conditions'. In E. Kahana, D.E. Biegel and M.L. Wykle (eds), *Family caregiving across the life-span*, pp. 331–55. California: Sage.

Keefe, J. and Fancey, P. (1997). 'Family visitation patterns: A Canadian perspective'. *Canadian Nursing Home* 8: 20–24.

————. (2000). 'The care continues: Responsibility for elderly relatives before and after admission to a long-term care facility'. *Family Relations* 49: 235–44.

Keith, C. (1995). 'Family caregiving systems: Models, resources and values'. *Journal of Marriage and the Family* 57: 179–89.

Kelly, J. and Sykes, P. (1989). 'Helping the helpers: A support group for family members of persons with AIDS'. *Social Work* 34: 239–42.

Koch, U., Harer, M., Jakob, U. and Siegrist, B. (1996). 'Parental reactions to cancer in their children'. In L. Baider, C.L. Cooper and A. Kaplan De-Nour (eds), *Cancer and the family*, pp. 149–72. Chichester: John Wiley.

Kramer, B.J. (1993a). 'The importance of relationship-focused coping strategies'. *Family Relations* 42: 383–91.

————. (1993b). 'Marital history and the prior relationships predictors of positive and negative outcomes among wife caregivers'. *Family Relations* 42: 367–75.

————. (2000). 'Husbands caring for wives with dementia'. *Health and Social Work* 25: 97–107.

Langan, T. (1970). 'The future of phenomenology'. In F.J. Smith (ed.), *Phenomenology in perspective*, pp. 1–15. The Hague: Martinus Nijhoff.

Langner, S.R. (1993). 'Ways of managing the experience of caregiving to elderly relatives'. *Western Journal of Nursing Research* 15: 582–94.

Lefley, H.P. (1996). *Family caregiving in mental illness*. California: Sage.

Lesar, S. and Maldonado, Y.A. (1997). 'The impact of children with HIV infection on the family system'. *Families in Societies* 78: 272–79.

Leserman, J., Perkins, D.O. and Evans, D.L. (1992). 'Coping with the threat of AIDS: The role of social support'. *American Journal of Psychiatry* 149: 1514–20.

Levine, C. (1994). 'AIDS and the changing concept of the family'. In R. Bor and J. Elford (eds), *The family and HIV*, pp. 3–22. London: Cassell.

Lippmann, S.B., James, W.A. and Frierson, R.L. (1993). 'AIDS and the family: Implication for counselling'. *AIDS Care* 5: 71–78.

Mane, P. (1995). *Behaviour change in the lives of women: Lessons learnt in the context of HIV/AIDS.* Geneva: UNAIDS.

McCann, T.V. (1999). 'Reluctance amongst nurses and doctors to care and treat patients with HIV/AIDS'. *AIDS Care* 11: 355–59.

McCann, K. and Wadsworth, E. (1994). 'The role of informal carers in supporting gay men who have HIV-related illness: What do they do and what are their needs?' In R. Bor and J. Elford (eds), *The family and HIV*, pp. 118–28. London: Cassell.

McDermott, S., Valentine, D., Anderson, D., Gallup, D. and Thompson, S. (1997). 'Parents of adults with mental retardation living in-home and out-home'. *American Journal of Orthopsychiatry* 67: 323–29.

McGrath, J.W., Ankrah, E.M., Schumann, D.A., Nkumbi, S. and Lubega, M. (1994). 'AIDS and the urban family: Its impact in Kampala, Uganda'. In R. Bor and J. Elford (eds), *The family and HIV*, pp. 208–28. London: Cassell.

Medalie, J. (1994). 'The caregiver as hidden patient'. In E. Kahana, D.E. Biegel and M.L. Winkle (eds), *Family caregiving across the lifespan*, pp. 312–30. California: Sage.

Midlarsky, E. (1994). 'Altruism through the life course'. In E. Kahana, D.E. Biegel and M.L. Winkle (eds), *Family caregiving across the lifespan*, pp. 69–95. California: Sage.

Miles, M.S. and Huberman, A.M. (1994). *Qualitative data analysis: A sourcebook of new methods.* California: Sage.

Miller, R. and Goldman, E. (1993). 'Counselling HIV infected women and families'. In M.A. Johnson and F.D. Johnstone (eds), *HIV infection in women*. London: Churchill Livingstone.

Milliken, P.J. and Northcott, H.C. (2003). 'Redefining parental identity: Caregiving and schizophrenia'. *Qualitative Health Research* 13: 100–13.

Millon, C., Mantero-Atienza, E. and Szapocznik, J. (1989). 'Psychological junctures in HIV infection'. In P. van Steijn (ed.), *AIDS: A combined environmental and systems approach*. Amsterdam: Swets & Zeitlinger.

Montgomery, R.J.V., Gonyea J.G. and Hooyman, N.R. (1985). 'Caregiving and the experience of subjective and objective burden'. *Family Relations* 34: 19–26.

Morse, J.M. (1991). 'Qualitative nursing research: A free-for-all?' In J.M. Morse (ed.), *Qualitative nursing research: A contemporary dialogue*, pp. 14–22. California: Sage.

Motenko, A.K. (1989). 'The frustrations, gratifications, and well-being of dementia caregivers'. *The Gerontologist* 29: 166–72.

National AIDS Control Organisation/NACO. (1998). 'Country scenario 1997–98'. New Delhi: NACO.

_____. (2001a). 'HIV Estimates for year 2001'. Retrieved 18 June 2003 from http://www.naco.nic.in/indianscene/esthiv.htm

_____. (2001b). 'Combating HIV/AIDS in INDIA 2000–2001'. Retrieved 18 June 2003 from http://www.naco.nic.in/indianscene/country.htm

Nelkin, D., Willis, D.P. and Parris, S.V. (1990). 'Introduction'. *Milbank Quarterly* 68 (Suppl): 1–9.

Neufeld, A. and Harrison, M.J. (1995). 'Reciprocity and social support in caregivers relationships: Variances and consequences'. *Qualitative Health Research* 5: 348–65.

New, M., Melvin, D. and Trickett, S. (1998). 'Community support to families living with HIV in London: An agency overview'. *AIDS Care* 10: 191–96.

Norbeck, J.S., Chafetz, L., Skodol-Wilson, H., Weiss, S.J. (1991). 'Social support needs of family caregivers of psychiatric patients from three age groups'. *Nursing Research* 40: 208–13.

Ntozi, J.P.M. (1997a). 'Effects of AIDS on children: The problem of orphans in Uganda'. *Health Transition Review* 7 (Suppl): 23–40.

_____. (1997b). 'AIDS morbidity and the role of the family in patient care in Uganda'. *Health Transition Review* 7 (Suppl): 1–22.

O'Donnell, M.C. (1992). 'Loss, grief and growth'. In M. Ross Seligson and K.E. Peterson (eds), *AIDS prevention and treatment: Hope, humour and healing*. New York: Hemisphere.

Orona, C.J. (1990). 'Temporality and identity loss due to Alzheimer's disease'. *Social Science and Medicine* 30: 1247–56.

Ostroff, J. and Steinglass, P. (1996). 'Psychosocial adaptation following treatment: A family systems perspective on childhood cancer survivorship'. In L. Baider, C.L. Cooper and A. Kaplan De-Nour (eds), *Cancer and the family*, pp. 129–48. Chichester: John Wiley.

Pai, S. and Kapur, R.L. (1981). 'Burden on the family of a psychiatric patient: Development of an interview schedule'. *British Journal of Psychiatry* 138: 332–740.

Paicheler, G. (1992). 'Society facing AIDS'. In M. Pollak (ed.), *AIDS: A problem of sociological research*, pp. 11–23. London: Sage.

Panda, S. (2002). 'The HIV/AIDS epidemic in India: An overview'. In S. Panda, A. Chatterjee and A.S. Abdul-Quader (eds), *Living with the AIDS virus*, pp. 17–35. New Delhi: Sage.

Parker, G. (1994). 'Spouse carers: Whose quality of life?'. In S. Baldwin, C. Godfrey and C. Propper (eds), *Quality of life*, pp. 120–30. London: Routledge.

Parks, S.H. and Pilisuk, M. (1991). 'Caregiver burden: Gender and the psychological costs of caregiving'. *American Journal of Orthopsychiatry* 61: 501–9.

Pierce, L.L. (2001). 'Caring and expressions of spirituality by urban caregivers of people with stroke in African American families'. *Qualitative Health Research* 11: 339–52.

Piercy, K.W. and Chapman, J.G. (2001). 'Adopting the caregiver role: A family legacy'. *Family Relations* 50: 386–93.

Pierret, J. (2000). 'Everyday life with AIDS/HIV: Surveys in the social sciences'. *Social Science and Medicine* 50: 1589–98.

Poindexter, C.C. and Linsk, N.L. (1998). 'Sources of support in a sample of HIV-affected older minority caregivers'. *Families in Society* 79: 491–503.

_____. (1999). 'HIV-related stigma in a sample of HIV-affected older female African-American caregivers'. *Social Work* 44: 46–61.

Pollak, M. (1992). 'Introduction'. In M. Pollak (ed.), *AIDS: A problem for sociological research*, pp. 1–9. London: Sage.

Poulshock, S.W. and Deimling, G.T. (1984). 'Families caring for elders in residence: Issues in the measurement of burden'. *Journal of Gerontology* 39: 230–39.

Powell-Cope, G.M. (1995). 'Experiences of gay couples affected by HIV infection'. *Qualitative Health Research* 5: 36–62

Powell-Cope, G.M. and Brown, M.A. (1992). 'Going public as an AIDS family caregiver'. *Social Science and Medicine* 34: 571–80.

Prabhu, K.S. (2000). 'Structural adjustment and health sector in India'. In M. Rao (ed.), *Disinvesting in health*, pp. 120–28. New Delhi: Sage.

Pratt, C.C., Schmall, V.L., Scott, W. and Cleland, M. (1985). 'Burden and coping strategies of caregivers to Alzheimer's patients'. *Family Relations* 34: 27–33.

Pruchno, R., Patrick, J.H. and Burant, C.J. (1997). 'African-American and white mothers of adults with chronic disabilities: Caregiving burden and satisfaction'. *Family Relations* 46: 335–46.

Pyke, K.D. and Bengston, V.L. (1996). 'Caring more or less: Individualistic and collectivist systems of family eldercare'. *Journal of Marriage and the Family* 58: 379–92.

Qadeer, I. (2000). 'The World Development Report, 1993: The brave new world of primary health care'. In M. Rao (ed.), *Disinvesting in health*, pp. 49–64. New Delhi: Sage.

Qureshi, H. and Walker, A. (1989). *The caring relationship: Elderly people and their families*. London: Macmillan.

Ramasubban, R. (1995). 'Patriarchy and the risks of STD and HIV transmission to women'. In M. Dasgupta, L.C. Chen and T.N. Krishnan (eds), *Women's health in India*, pp. 212–44. Bombay: Oxford University Press.

—————. (1998). 'HIV/AIDS in India: Gulf between rhetoric and reality'. *Economic and Political Weekly* 33: 2865–72.

Rawat, D.S. (1999). 'Living with HIV/AIDS is not easy'. *AIDS Research and Review* 2: 50–52.

Ray, M.A. (1994). 'The richness of phenomenology: Philosophic, theoretic and methodologic concerns'. In J.M. Morse (ed.), *Critical issues in qualitative research methods*, pp. 117–33. California: Sage.

Reidy, M., Taggart, M.E. and Asselin, L. (1994). 'Psychosocial needs expressed by natural caregivers of HIV infected children'. In R. Bor and J. Elford (eds), *The family and HIV*, pp. 169–86. London: Cassell.

Roberto, K.A. (1993). 'Older caregivers of family members with developmental disabilities: Changes in roles and perceptions'. In K.A. Roberto (ed.), *The elderly caregiver: Caring for adults with developmental disabilities*, pp. 39–50. Newbury Park, California: Sage.

Ross, M.M., Rosenthal, C.J. and Dawson, P. (1997). 'Spousal caregiving in the institutional setting: Task performance'. *Canadian Journal on Aging* 16: 51–69.

Roychaudhuri, J., Mondal, D., Boral, A. and Bhattacharya, D. (1995). 'Family among long-term psychiatric patients'. *Indian Journal of Psychiatry* 37: 81–85.

Sabhesan, S. (1991). 'Families of patients neuropsychologically handicapped after head injury'. In M. Desai (ed.), *Research on families with problems in India* Vol. II. Bombay: TISS.

Sathiamoorthy, K. and Solomon, S. (1997). 'Socio-economic realities of living with HIV'. In P. Godwin (ed.), *Socio-economic implications of the epidemic*. New Delhi: UNDP.

Scharlach, A.E. (1994). 'Caregiving and employment: Competing or complementary roles'. *The Gerontologist* 29: 382–87.

Schwandt, T.A. (1997). *Qualitative inquiry: A dictionary of terms.* California: Sage.

Seeley, J., Kajura, E., Bachengana, C., Okongo, M., Wagner, U. and Mulder, D.
(1994). 'The extended family and support for people with AIDS in a rural
population in South West Uganda: A safety net with holes?'. In R. Bor and
J. Elford (eds.), *The family and HIV,* pp. 141–50. London: Cassell.

Seltzer, M.M. and Heller, T. (1997). 'Families and caregiving across the life-
course: Research advances on the influence of context'. *Family Relations* 46:
321–23.

Sequeira, E.M., Rao, P.M., Subbakrishna, D.K. and Prabhu, G.G. (1990). 'Perceived burden and coping styles of the mothers of mentally handicapped
children'. *NIMHANS Journal* 8: 63–68.

Sethi, G. (1999). 'Government response to HIV/AIDS'. In S. Pachauri (ed.),
Implementing a reproductive health agenda in India: A beginning, pp. 389–413.
New Delhi: Population Council.

—————. (2002). 'AIDS in India: The government's response'. In S. Panda, A.
Chatterjee and A.S. Abdul-Quader (eds), *Living with the AIDS virus,* pp. 36–
61. New Delhi: Sage.

Sewpaul, V. and Mahlalela, T. (1998). 'When both mother and baby are HIV
positive: Psychosocial implications for black women in South African society'. Paper presented at the Joint World Congress of the International
Association of Schools of Social Work and the International Federation of
Social Workers—Jerusalem, 5–9 July.

Shagle, S. (1995). 'A view into the family and social life in India'. *Family Perspective* 29: 423–46.

Shah, A.M. (1999). 'Changes in the family and the elderly'. *Economic and
Political Weekly* 34: 1179–82.

Shaw, S.H. (1992). 'Psychotherapy of the HIV positive patient and the family:
An integrated approach'. In P.I. Ahmed (ed.), *Living and dying with AIDS,* pp.
87–101. New York: Plenum.

Sheehan, N.W. and Nuttall, P. (1988). 'Conflict, emotion and personal strain
among family caregivers'. *Family Relations* 37: 92–98.

Sherr, L. (1993). 'Discordant couples'. In L. Sherr (ed.), *AIDS and the heterosexual
population.* Switzerland: Harwood.

Shields, C.G. (1992). 'Family interaction and caregivers of Alzheimer's disease
patients'. *Family Process* 31: 19–33.

Singhanetra-Renard, A., Chongsatitmun, C. and Wibulswasdi, P. (1996). *Household and community responses to HIV/AIDS in Thailand.* Unpublished project
report. Chiang Mai: Chiang Mai University.

Smith, K. (1989). 'Non-governmental organisations in the health field: Col-
laboration, integration and contrasting aims'. *Social Science and Medicine*
29: 395–402.

Sohier, R. (1993). 'Filial reconstruction: A theory of development through
adversity'. *Qualitative Health Research* 3: 465–92.

Solomon, S., Kumaraswamy, N., Ganesh, A.K. and Amalraj, R.E. (1998). 'Prevalence and risk factors of HIV-1 and HIV-2 infection in urban and rural areas
in Tamil Nadu, India'. *International Journal of STD and AIDS* 9: 98–103.

Songwathana, P. and Manderson, L. (1998). 'Perceptions of HIV/AIDS and caring for people with terminal AIDS in Southern Thailand'. *AIDS Care* 10 (Suppl 2): S155–65.

Sosnowitz, B.G. and Kovacs, D.R. (1992). 'From burying to caring: Family AIDS support groups'. In J. Huber and B. Schneider (eds), *The social context of AIDS*, pp. 131–44. California: Sage.

Spiegelberg, H. (1982). *The phenomenologic movement: A historical introduction.* The Hague: Martinus Nijhoff.

Srinivas, S. (1978). *The changing position of Indian women.* Delhi: Oxford University Press.

Stein, J., Steinberg, M., Allwood, C., Karstaedt, A. and Brouard, P. (1997). 'Nurse-counsellors' perceptions regarding HIV/AIDS counselling objectives at Baragwanath Hospital, Soweto'. In J. Catalan, L. Sherr and B. Hedge (eds), *The impact of AIDS*, pp. 191–98. Netherlands: Harwood.

Stephenson, J.S. (1985). *Death, grief and mourning.* USA: Free Press.

Teguis, A. (1992). 'Dying with AIDS'. In P.I. Ahmed (ed.) *Living and dying with AIDS*, pp.153–75. New York: Plenum.

Teguis, A. and Ahmed, P.I. (1992). 'Living with AIDS: An overview'. In P.I. Ahmed (ed.), *Living and dying with AIDS*, pp. 7–17. New York: Plenum.

Theorell, T., Blomkvist, V., Jonsson, H., Schulman, S., Berntorp, E. and Stigendal, L. (1995). 'Social support and the development of immune function in human immunodeficiency virus'. *Psychosomatic Medicine* 57: 32–36.

Thomas, G., Sinha, N.P. and Thomas, J.K. (1997). *AIDS, social work and the law.* New Delhi: Rawat.

Thomson, K. (1994). 'Being positive'. In J. Bury (ed.), *Working with women and AIDS.* London: Routledge.

Townsend, A.L. and Franks, M.M. (1997). 'Quality of relationship between elderly spouses: Influence on spouse caregivers' subjective effectiveness'. *Family Relations* 46: 33–39.

Traustadottir, R. (1991). 'Mothers who care: Gender, disability, and family life'. *Journal of Family Issues* 12: 211–18.

Tuck, I., du-Mont, P., Evans, G. and Shupe, J. (1997). 'The experience of caring for an adult child with schizophrenia'. *Archives of Psychiatric Nursing* 11: 118–25.

Tulsidhar, V.B. (1993). 'Expenditure compression and health sector outlays'. *Economic and Political Weekly* 28: 2473–77.

Twigg, J. and Atkin, K. (1994). *Carers perceived: Policy and practices in informal care.* Buckingham, UK: Open University Press.

UNAIDS [Joint United Nations Programme on HIV/AIDS]. (2000). *Caring for carers.* Geneva: UNAIDS

————. (2001a). *Investing in our future: Psychosocial support affected by HIV/AIDS.* Geneva: UNAIDS.

————. (2001b). *Parents providing care to adult sons and daughters with HIV/AIDS in Thailand.* Geneva: UNAIDS

————. (2002). *Report on the global HIV/AIDS epidemic 2002.* Geneva: UNAIDS. Retrieved 20 November 2002 from http://www.unaids.org/barcelona,%20report/global_estimate.pdf

UNAIDS/UNICEF/USAID [Joint United Nations Programme for HIV/AIDS/United Nations Children's Fund/United States Agency for International Development]. (2002). *Children on the brink 2002.* Washington DC: TvT.

van Manen, M. (1998). *Researching lived experience*. Canada: Althouse.

Verma, R.K., Bhende, A.A. and Mane, P. (1999). 'NGO response to HIV/AIDS: A focus on women'. In S. Pachauri (ed.), *Implementing a reproductive health agenda in India: A beginning*, pp. 415–33. New Delhi: Population Council.

Verma, R.K. and Roy, T.K. (2002). 'HIV risk behaviour and the sociocultural environment'. In S. Panda, A. Chatterjee and A.S. Abdul-Quader (eds), *Living with the AIDS virus*, pp. 77–90. New Delhi: Sage.

Waerness, K. (1985). 'Informal and formal care in old age: What is wrong with the new ideology of community care in the Scandinavian welfare state today'. Paper presented at the Conference on Gender Division and Policies for Community Care, University of Kent, Canterbury, UK.

Walker, A.J., Pratt, C.C. and Eddy, L. (1995). 'Informal caregiving to aging family members'. *Family Relations* 44: 402–41.

Walker, A.J., Pratt, C.C. and Oppy, N.C. (1992). 'Perceived reciprocity in family caregiving'. *Family Relations* 41: 82–85.

Wiener, L., Theut, S., Steinberg, S.M., Riekert, K.A. and Pizzo, P.A. (1994). 'The HIV infected child: Parental responses and psychosocial implications'. *American Journal of Orthopsychiatry* 64: 485–92.

Wight, R.G. (2000). 'Precursive depression among HIV infected AIDS caregivers over time'. *Social Science and Medicine* 51: 759–70.

Wilson, J. (1994). 'Women as carers'. In J. Bury (ed.), *Working with women and AIDS*. London: Routledge.

World Bank. (1993). *World development report*. Oxford: Oxford University Press.

Wrubel, J. and Folkman, S. (1997). 'What informal caregivers actually do: The caregiving skills of partners of men with AIDS'. *AIDS Care* 9: 691–706.

Yaima, N., Nigthouja, S., Sharma, D., Bijaya, L., Shyamkanhai, K., Narendra, P., Lisam, K. and Agarwal, K. (1997). 'Lessons from home-based care for persons affecting with HIV and AIDS'. In O.P. Aggarwal, A.K. Sharma and A. Indrayan (eds.), *HIV/AIDS research in India*. New Delhi: NACO.

Young, R.F. and Kahana, E. (1994). 'Caregiving issues after a heart attack'. In E. Kahana, D.E. Biegel and M.L. Wykle (eds), *Family caregiving across the lifespan*, pp. 262–86. California: Sage.

Index

Abel, E.K., 21
activities of daily living (ADL), 25
adolescent, caregiver, 70; children, 151, 154
Agarwal, B., 187, 188
ageing parental caregiver, 19
AIDS, 42, 49, 51, 58, 59, 64, 65, 70, 93–95, 110, 113, 115, 132, 142, 144, 155, 162, 163, 170–172, 177, 184, 195; research, 43; affected individuals, 44; care, 47; test, 92; buddies, 59; service organisations, 60; patients, 61, 64; information, 64; related stigma, 70, 193; treatment of, 71; transmission of, 64; legislation, 194; educators, 194; epidemic, 193
AIDS-related complex (ARC), 62
allopathic systems, 200
allopathy, 96
alternative system(s), 200; of medicine, 97, 199
Altman, D., 196
Alzheimer's dementia (AD), 24, 25, 27, 29, 32, 33, 192
Andhra Pradesh, 43
Ankrah, E.M., 63, 70
antenatal care, 157, 158
anti-retroviral(s), 199; treatment, 89, 119, 126
Archbold, P.G., 27
Arunachal Pradesh, 43
Assam, 43

Ayurveda, 200

Barber, C.E., 23
Barbour, R.S., 195, 196
Bastardo, Y.M. and Kimberlin, C.L., 183
Bengston, V.L. and Roberts, R.E., 36
Berg-Weger, M., 28
Bharat, S. and Aggleton, P., 60, 61
Bharat, S., 60–62, 67, 71, 191, 192, 195–97
Bishop, A. and Scudder, J., 75
Blieszner, R. and Shifflet, P.A., 32
Bombay Metropolitan Region Development Authority (BMRDA), 80n
Brouwer, C.N.M., 52, 53
Brown, M.A. and Seltz, K., 12, 13
buddy systems, 59–60
Bulger, M.W., 28
burnout, 56, 70, 72

Campbell, C.A., 52, 55
caregiving, husbands, 11, 25; mother(s), 12, 110, 116, 120; wives, 12, 25, 84; family, 11; relationship, 31; experience, 22, 26; spouse, 26; women, 102; terminal stage, 51; doctor, 127
caregiver wives, 28
caregiver–care receiver, relationship, 26, 27, 28, 30, 31, 32, 33, 70, 73, 192; dyad, 38; relations, 31, 192; interactions, 37, 192

Chatterjee, M., 197
Chesla, C.A., 32, 33
child/ren caregiver(s), 47, 54, 191;
    in HIV/AIDS, 53, 54
Cipla, 199
clinical, care, 68; treatment, 98
collectivism, 15
commercial sex worker (CSW), 43,
    64, 192
community care, 14, 199; policies
    of, 45, 182; programmes, 59
condoms, 189
confidentiality, 92, 116, 196; issues
    of, 92; breach of, 195; violations
    of, 158, 165
conflicted care, 34
Conger C.O. and Marshall, E.S., 27,
    31
counselling, 71, 183–85
Cowles, V.K. and Rodgers, B.L., 72
Creswell, J.W., 75
Crockner, J. and Quinn, D.M., 193

D'Cruz, P., 55, 62, 66, 190, 191, 197
deinstitutionalisation movement,
    182
dementia, 33
denial, 22, 72
depression, 24, 26, 72
Desai, K.G. and Naik, R.D., 190
discrimination, 66, 159, 164, 180, 196
discriminatory, responses, 195;
    care, 195; treatment, 195
distanced care, 34
Douglass, 35
drug Ab/use, 91, 195
Drug Rehabilitation Centre, 86
Dwyer, J. W. and Coward, R.T., 25

elderly caregivers, 56, 121, 190, 191
emotional, support, 12, 68, 98, 106,
    166, 168, 175, 178, 179, 182–84,
    189; care, 164; support pro-
    grammes, 185; distress, 41, 152
engaged care, 33, 53
eunuchs, 192
extended family, 68; care, 53

family caregiver, 70, 72, 199
feminisation of, caregiving, 15;
    care, 16; poverty, 188
Ferree, 17
filial caregiver, 20, 26
Folbre, 188

gay related immune disorder
    (GRID), 59
gay, couples, 58; men, 59;
    seropositives, 59; community,
    59; seropositive individuals, 73
gender(s), 15, 16, 17, 61, 62, 188,
    189; theory, 16, 17; differences,
    25; differences in caregiving,
    16; -based inequities, 17;
    equality, 187; power differen-
    tials, 189; role socialisation, 188
geriatric population, 19
Given, C.W. and Given, B.A., 12,
    21, 37
Glover, L. and Miller, D., 184, 192
Gorna, R., 189
Graham, H., 11
grandparents, caregiver, 55, 57,
Grunseit, A. and Kippax, S., 195

Hackl, K.L., 48, 195, 196
haemophilia, 51, 52
Haley, W.E. and Pardo, K.M., 29
hands-on, care, 68, 110, 136;
    physical care, 141
health management, 61
healthcare, 71; advocacy, 68;
    agencies, 92; system, 92, 96,
    107, 121, 122, 157, 165, 196,
    198; professionals, 92; facilities,
    147; centres, 165; workers, 195,
    196, 198; intervention, 162;
    doctor, 169; security, 184;
    standards, 198
health-related quality of life
    (HRQL), 183
Heidegger, 75
Heller, T., 29
Herek, G.M., 193
Herek, G.M. and Mitnick, L., 193

hermeneutic, phenomenological approach, 182; phenomenology, 77; conversations, 85
heterosexual transmission, 44, 188
high risk behaviour, 44
highly active anti-retroviral treatment (HAART), 199
high-tech nursing, 68
Himmelweit, 192
Hirschfeld, M., 33
HIV, 42, 47, 49, 50, 52, 56, 63–65, 68, 70, 82, 99, 100, 104, 110, 113, 120, 122, 123, 134, 184, 193, 198; pandemic, 81; related treatment, 138, 149, 158; related services, 162; seropositive participants, 96; infection(s), 44, 62, 66, 103, 107, 113, 116, 118, 123, 134, 137, 156, 190, 198; transmission, 44, 64, 70; status disclosure, 48; status, 88, 114, 137; diagnosis, 49, 66, 94, 95, 113, 155, 184; prevention information, 49; treatment, 49; virus, 43, 89; infected gay caregiver, 58; negative gay caregiver, 58; affected caregiver, 66; related stigma, 66; related needs, 66; risk reduction changes, 189; testing, 157; treatment, 194; seropositive individuals, 194; positive, 43, 51, 133, 135;— children, 47; child, 52; women caregivers, 48; gays, 70; caregiver, 58, 107; people, 79, 86, 164, 195; person, 92, 159; family member, 99; status, 112; individual, 63; infected;— women, 48; children, 53; parents, 53; individual(s), 60, 95, 194; people, 65, 183; care-recipient, 65; person, 72
HIV/AIDS, 14, 43, 45, 46, 47, 53–57, 59–61, 63, 68, 70–73, 75, 97, 127, 140, 150, 155, 157, 163, 165, 166, 181, 182, 188, 190–98; related services, 44; related

service organisation, 196; residential facility for, 98; people living with, 72; research, 80; awareness programmes, 194; attitudes towards, 196; humanistic policies on, 194
homoeopathic services, 97; medicines, 97
homoeopathy, 200
homophobia, 195
homosexual(s), 50, 64, 192
Hooyman, N.R. and Gonyea, J., 22, 24, 25
hospice home care, 30
Household (HH), 12, 47, 60–63, 71, 111; chores, 49; tasks, 60, 150
Hull, M.M., 30
Husserl, 75

illiteracy, 44
individualism, 15, 190
instrumental activities of daily living (IADL), 25; care, 29
insurance, 197; agencies, 13
interpretive sociology, 74
intravenous drug use/rs (IVDUs), 44, 50, 64, 86, 192

Jeon, Y.H. and Madjar, I., 29

Karnataka, 43
Kazak, A.E. and Christakis, D.A., 37
Keith, C., 17
Kelly, J. and Sykes, P., 72
kinship caregiver, 55, 56
Kramer, B.J., 23, 26

Langner, S.R., 30
Lesar, S. and Maldonado, Y.A., 53
London, 54
long-term care (LTC), 25; facility, 40; long-term institutionalisation, 14

Madras, 43
Maharashtra, 43
managed care, 34
Manipur, 43

marginalised, households, 54;
   groups, 73, 192
McCann, T.V., 195
Medalie, J., 27
medical support, 98
Meghalaya, 43
middle-aged caregivers, 41
Midlarsky, E., 34
migratory patterns, 44
Million, C., 63, 184
mortality rate, 183
Motenko, A.K., 28
multiple, caregiver, 21; infections, 56
Mumbai, 80, 96, 113, 147, 148, 150,
   158, 159, 163, 171, 172, 176,
   178, 182
mutual monogamy, 189

NACO, 43
network support, 98
Neufeld, A. and Harrison, M.J., 34
NGO, 82, 93, 98–100, 111, 117, 118,
   121, 123–26, 136, 139, 142, 146,
   153, 157, 160, 164, 166, 167,
   177, 181, 197; centres, 95
Norbeck, J.S., 29
Ntozi, J.P.M., 68
nuclear, households, 137;
family/ies, 53, 147

opportunistic infection, 80; of TB, 98
Orona, C.J., 33
ostracism, 49, 66

pandemic, 42, 45, 46, 182, 198
parental caregiver, 18, 19, 51, 52, 109
Parker, G., 18
Parks, S.H. and Pilisuk, M., 23, 25
patriarchal society, 132
paediatric, AIDS, 44, 51, 52; HIV, 51
phenomenological, 22; tradition,
   75; study, 78; reflection, 83;
   approach, 183
phenomenology, 74, 75, 77, 78
Pierce, L.L., 29
Piercy, K.W. and Chapman, J.G., 15
Poindexter, C.C. and Linsk, N.L.,
   65, 66

post-death phase, 145, 147, 178, 179
post-positivist epistemology, 74
poverty, 44, 52
predictive medicine, 42
primary caregiver, 15, 17, 19, 39,
   50, 53, 60, 68, 72, 112
primary prevention, 45
private health sector, 95, 196, 198;
   healthcare intervention, 162;
   doctor, 169; nursing home, 95,
   159, 160
professional caregiver, 60
promiscuity, 63; sexual, 195
prostitution, 195
psychoneuroimmunology, 183
public, health sector, 95, 196,
   198; -sector hospital, 93, 95, 158;
   hospital(s), 149, 158, 159, 162,
   164; health centres, 96, 97
Pyke, K.D. and Bengston, V.L., 15

quacks, 200
Qureshi, H. and Walker A., 20

Rajasthan, 43
reciprocity, 34, 35, 37, 65, 106, 128,
   192
residential care, 86, 100; facility,
   124, 126
Roberto, K.A., 28

Scharlach, A.E., 28
schizophrenia, 28
secondary prevention, 45
Seeley, J., 63, 66
Seltzer, M.M. and Heller, T., 24, 182
Sen, Amartya, 187
seronegative, 62; caregivers, 57,
   84, 85, 107; brother, 111
seropositive/ity/s, 43, 44, 48, 53,
   56, 157, 159, 176, 179, 189;
   person, 57, 61; people, 60, 183,
   196; status, 50, 72, 94, 130;
   diagnosis, 52, 86, 88, 92, 101,
   111, 114, 132, 134, 158, 170,
   178; parents, 54, 55;
   individual(s), 65, 70, 80, 88, 104,
   165, 184, 196; caregiving wives,

84; caregiving groups, 191; husbands, 130; person, 98, 163; family member, 125; women, 130, 189, 190; member, 182; caregiver, 81, 85; wives, 183
Sewpaul, V. and Mahlalela, T., 50, 52, 195
sexually transmitted disease (STD), 44
Shah, A.M., 190
Shaw, S.H., 184
Sheehan, N.W. and Nuttall, P., 23
Sikkim, 43
single parent caregiver, 19
skip-generation parenting, 53, 56–57
social exchange theory, 21
social, network, 113, 118, 140, 157, 158, 193, 196; support, 183; system, 59, 94
Sohier, R., 59
spirituality, 30, 66
spousal caregiver, 18, 26
Srinivas, S., 185
stigma, 24, 56, 58, 69, 81, 92, 120, 123, 137, 190, 193, 196
stress, 25, 69
structural adjustment programme (SAP), 182, 197
suicide, 49
support group, 71

Tamil Nadu, 43

Tanzania, 55
Teguis, A. and Ahmed, P.I., 184
tertiary prevention, 45
Thailand, 50, 51, 62
thalassemia, 52, 113, 120, 122
Thompson, K., 16, 195
traditional, caregivers, 47; healers, 51
Traustadottir, R., 11
tuberculosis (TB), 98, 99, 113, 114, 125, 165, 178, 180

UNAIDS, 43, 55
United States, 59

Van Manen, M., 77–79, 83, 85, 182
Venezuela, 183
vertical transmission, 44
voluntary, sector, 97, 124, 196–98; organisation(s), 124, 135; caregiver, 59

Waerness, K., 11
Walker A.J., 11, 12, 16, 36
Wight, R.G., 58
World Bank, 197
Wrubel, J. and Folkman, S., 60, 68, 69, 70

Young, R.F. and Kahana, E., 37

Zimbabwe, 55, 61

The Author

Premilla D'Cruz is currently Assistant Professor, Organizational Behaviour, at the Indian Institute of Management Kozhikode. She was previously on the Faculty of the Indian Institute of Technology, Kanpur, besides having worked at the Tata Institute of Social Sciences, Mumbai, from where she obtained her Ph.D. Her research interests include gender, creativity, emotion, health studies, information and communication technologies and organisational life, family psychology and qualitative research methods. In addition to numerous journal articles, Dr D'Cruz has previously published *In Sickness and in Health*.